THE *Yoga-Sūtra* OF PATAÑJALI

THE *Yoga-Sūtra* OF PATAÑJALI

A New Translation with Commentary

CHIP HARTRANFT

SHAMBHALA
Boulder
2003

Shambhala Publications, Inc.
4720 Walnut Street
Boulder, Colorado 80301
www.shambhala.com

20 19 18 17 16 15 14 13

Printed in the United States of America
♾ This edition is printed on acid-free paper that meets the American National Standards Institute Z39.48 Standard.
♻ This book is printed on 30% postconsumer recycled paper.
For more information please visit www.shambhala.com.
Distributed in the United States by Penguin Random House LLC and in Canada by Random House of Canada Ltd

Designed by Ruth Kolbert

Library of Congress Cataloging-in-Publication Data
Patañjali.
[Yogasutra. English & Sanskrit]
The Yoga-Sutra of Patañjali: a new translation with commentary/Chip Hartranft.
p. cm. —(Shambhala classics)
Includes bibliographical references.
ISBN 978-1-59030-023-7
1. Yoga—Early works to 1800. I. Hartranft, Chip. II. Title. III. Series.
B132.Y6P24313 2003
181'.452—dc21
2002026877

To Patañjali and Siddhartha Gautama,
"spiritual physicians" to humanity,
and to Didi, who is mine

Contents

INTRODUCTION

THE *YOGA-SŪTRA* OF PATAÑJALI IS ONE OF THE MOST enlightening spiritual documents of all time. Nearly two thousand years old, this collection of 196 compact observations on the nature of consciousness and liberation remains unrivaled for its penetrating insight. Though brief, the *Yoga-Sūtra* manages to cut to the heart of the human dilemma. With uncommon directness, Patañjali analyzes how we know what we know and why we suffer. He then provides a meditative program through which each of us can fulfill the primary purposes of consciousness: to see things as they are and to achieve freedom from suffering. Weaving the threads of ancient yogic knowledge into a detailed map of human possibility, the *Yoga-Sūtra* stands as a testament to heroic self-awareness, defining yoga for all time.

Even today, from a distance of two millennia, we can be sure that Patañjali's inward quest arose from a deeply ingrained desire to extract happiness and meaning from the mysteries of life, consciousness, and mortality. Such a desire has been universal among humans of all cultures since prehistory, and it resonates in us as strongly today as ever. In fact, yoga now enjoys an unprecedented and ever growing popularity in East and West. Just as Western thought and technology have crossed geographical borders and found a home in India, Indian thought long ago migrated throughout Southeast Asia, China, and Japan, profoundly enriching the cultures of each region, and has continued to spread across the globe. Today the central themes of Indian thought, especially regarding consciousness, continue to penetrate both Asian and Western worlds of art, philosophy, and spirituality, providing a much-needed counterbalance to Western orthodoxies. These patterns of cross-fertilization reflect a universality that labels like "Indian" and "Western" obscure.

However, most of the yoga practiced worldwide today would be unrecognizable to earlier yogis like Patañjali who attained realization in meditative stillness. Had he lived some seven centuries later, in the tenth century instead of the third, his system might well have incorporated movements from the leading form of yoga now practiced, hatha yoga, which was developed in part to temper the bodymind and focus its energies for meditation. In Patañjali's era, though, the yoga posture, or *āsana,* was simply a means of sitting as steadily and effortlessly as possible and was not an exercise system of any kind. This older, contemplative yoga has come to be known as *rāja-yoga*—the "royal" or "exalted" path—distinguishing it from the later hatha yoga. It is also often referred to as classical yoga for the same reason. The yoga of Patañjali is a process of stilling and interiorization, in which utter physical and mental calm is brought to every aspect of human personhood and experience. For him, *āsana* was but the bodily aspect of this process.

Indeed, when Patañjali uses the word *yoga,* he means "yoking." Its root, *yuj,* is a direct forerunner of the modern word *yoke.* The practice of yoga is meant to rein in the tendency of consciousness to gravitate toward external things, to identify with them and try to locate happiness in them. Steady practice at "yoking" teaches consciousness how to turn inward toward itself and realize the true nature of its underlying awareness. Only then, he assures us, can we understand why we are alive, why we suffer, and how we might become happy and wise.

The experience of realization is not altogether unfamiliar to us. Most of us have had flashes of enlightenment at one time or another, usually when we find ourselves caught up in an absorbing event. At profound moments of engagement—a sunrise, birth, wedding, or death—time seems to stand still and awareness grows spacious and inclusive. For a momentless moment, it feels as if we are seeing directly into the nature of things.

Unfortunately, insight of this kind is a serendipity, more *given* than willed, and usually passes quickly. One of the profound wisdoms of the yoga tradition, though, is the recognition that the capacity to see into the nature of things is intrinsic. The yoking practice of yoga arose as human beings actively sought to harness this faculty. While realization always has a spontaneous, unwilled quality, systematic practice at stilling the body and mind through yoga makes it far more likely that we can enter—and eventually abide in—this kind of deep, absorptive knowing.

Prakṛti and Puruṣa

From Patañjali's perspective, most physical and mental actions arise from a fundamental misunderstanding of reality and therefore entail suffering. Everything that exists in creation, he explains, is different from pure awareness. This includes not only the body and its sense organs but also consciousness and its contents, such as sensation, thought, emotional feeling, and memory. Therefore, everything that we might think of as *me*—physical, emotional, conceptual, spiritual, internal, external—is part of nature, or *prakṛti*. In this view, all of *me*, even the innermost part, is material stuff, impermanent, and subject to cause and effect. Some of the stuff that *me* comprises is subtle, for example, the recognition of a familiar taste like an apple. Some of it is gross, such as the teeth that are chewing it. But all of oneself is *prakṛti*.

Pure awareness, on the other hand, is not stuff of any sort and is therefore free of cause and effect. It was never created and never ends, existing beyond time. Even to use the word *it* or assert that "it exists" lends pure awareness a seeming substantiality it does not possess. Because it is immaterial, it has no location, movement, or other natural properties; nor does it have anything in common with consciousness or thought, other than the role of observing them. It is literally intangible, impersonal, and inconceivable.

In Patañjali's view, pure awareness, or *puruṣa,* is what actually sees creation unfolding, primarily on a screen we call consciousness. The screen of consciousness is the foundation of human experience, a part of the phenomenal world it represents, and under ordinary circumstances it actually feels like the subjective "eye" that is observing everything. In Patañjali's view, though, no aspect of creation, including consciousness, can see itself, because it is material stuff. In the same way that a television cannot view its own programs, consciousness requires a witnessing awareness. Indeed, just as the television exists not for its own sake but for the viewer, consciousness is at the disposal of pure awareness.

However, according to the *Yoga-Sūtra,* under ordinary circumstances pure awareness has no sense of itself at all. Immaterial, unmoving, nonconceptual, it is completely submerged beneath the waves of consciousness. Like the rest of nature's stuff, consciousness is embroiled in an ongoing process of creation, spiraling from form to form, pattern to pattern. This incessant repatterning of consciousness distorts its actual relationship to pure awareness. Although pure awareness is unchanging, its lack of substance or motion renders it invisible to consciousness. After all, the contents of consciousness—perception, thought, memory—are made of stuff and arise from material transformations. Because of these attributes, consciousness is an instrument poorly suited to detect the pure awareness that is watching it. In other words, consciousness is a thing that is only good at showing things.

Like the rest of creation, the aspect that Patañjali calls consciousness, or *citta,* is evolving. Its evolutionary goal is to refine itself to the point where it can become so still, unmoving, and equally absorbed in all phenomena that it becomes very much like pure awareness itself. In that instant, it can reflect pure awareness back to itself, making it realize that it is distinct and separate from nature. In other words, the underlying purpose of creation is to reveal pure seeing to itself.

MOTION AND STILLNESS

All the contents of creation that Patañjali can observe—including his body, senses, and mind—appear volatile. No matter what aspect of nature he selects as an object of contemplation, he notices before long that the object's fundamental properties—light, mass, motion—are actually a sequence of transformations and changing proportions. By calmly and patiently observing the play of sensation, thought, and feeling as he trains attention on some kind of object, he has come to the conclusion that this play includes both the things of the world and his consciousness of them, and never stops.

Consciousness behaves something like water in the ocean. As its currents stir the water into waves, the water's surface is set in motion. When this occurs, two essential properties of water become invisible—it ceases to appear either transparent or reflective. Instead, its agitations disrupt the surface, fragmenting the reflected light and rendering the surface opaque. If Patañjali had used the image of water, he might have pointed to the two ways one again comes to see its essential transparency and reflection. The first way is to make the water *still,* and the second is to move from the surface inward—*interiorization.*

Instead of water, Patañjali uses the metaphor of consciousness becoming a transparent jewel that mirrors everything before awareness—the object, or thing one is looking at; the subject, or sense of "me" watching; and the sense of relationship between subject and object that we generally take to be perceiving itself. In the mirror of this reflective state, called coalescence, awareness recognizes that all things—and the consciousness representing them—are made of the same stuff.

Paradoxically, as one begins to recognize the unity of all things and their separateness from awareness, one can also see the nature of their transformations more clearly. While pure awareness is unchanging and exists beyond time, the stuff of creation is undergoing constant change, instant by instant. Patañjali recognized that one of the most primary internal forces in a human being is the inclination toward selfhood. Self-making has the effect of organizing the shifting contents of consciousness into a seamless pseudo-reality that seems to unfold over time. This constructed reality consists of oneself as subject and everything else as the object. From this vantage point, the world and the self feel like enduring entities, each different from the other, with essential qualities that are carried forward through time.

The self is remarkably successful at maintaining this perspective—under ordinary conditions, we are simply incapable of seeing ourselves as other than a singular entity. At any given moment we live and operate from the conviction that we are the same person who was born some years ago and has had a continuous life right up to the present. In fact, not just our own person but all objects seem to have an essential reality of their own. A clay pot is imbued with "potness" despite the fact that its identity as a pot is but a momentary way station between coming from the earth and returning to it.

However, when consciousness becomes truly motionless, these appearances of permanence and continuity break down. Just as turbulent water's opacity gives way to transparency when it calms, the illusory reality represented in consciousness becomes transparent as body and mind grow deeply still.

Another perceptual change occurs during this process. One's sense of time becomes spacious, with consciousness sensing many more individual events than before and beginning to perceive its own workings in more detail. What had seemed like a smooth flow—the reality of the phenomenal world—can now be seen as the flickering of microphenomena arising and vanishing with unimaginable speed and subtlety. Under ordinary circumstances they had blended together something like the individual frames in a motion picture, giving the illusion of solidity and continuity. As this illusion falls apart, the self and the world reveal themselves to be nothing but a stream of rapidly changing events. Where earlier they had seemed solid enough to endure through time, now they can be seen as piecemeal and temporary. In this light, the dramas of consciousness no longer seem real, nor do they propel one any longer toward thoughts or actions that will bring more suffering. One recognizes, at last, that the unchanging awareness that knows this reality is the true center of human existence and that it is free of suffering.

EFFORT AND EFFORTLESSNESS

In order to still the movements of consciousness to the point of realization—seeing reality as it is—we must allow each aspect of ourselves to clarify. Patañjali's program of clarification involves "yoking," or sublimating all our energies to the process of awakening. Each part of this program, although interdependent with every other part, addresses a different level of personhood. We are encouraged to bring clarity to our relationships with the beings and objects of the external world, so that those relationships might cease to generate suffering or impede realization. Likewise, we are assured that a disciplined inner life is the most direct path to happiness. Our bodyminds can know their true nature by letting themselves gravitate toward effortless sitting and breathing. And our attention can be stabilized, with perception coming to rest in the present moment and clarifying to the point where the unity of all things is known beyond argument or reservation.

In every domain of personhood, therefore, we must make an effort to bring about the yogic transformation. However, in Patañjali's view the commotion of our ordinary physical and mental life conceals the fact that our thoughts and actions are almost always tinged with wanting, aversion, egoism, or fear of extinction. Thus, as we settle into the stilling process, or *nirodha,* we come to recognize that these energies of suffering are the sparks quickening every part of our inner landscape into action. This includes even our efforts to transcend them through yoga. No matter how deep our sincerity or robust our desire to awaken, we cannot move very far toward clarity before certain of our efforts themselves become obstacles on our path.

Patañjali's program of moral and personal discipline can seem impossibly difficult at first. The challenge lies not in the prescription itself, though, but in overcoming the well-established mental and physical habits that already produce suffering in our lives. These habits of perception and behavior cost us dearly, yet we cannot help but hold them dear, for they *are* us. That is, we have all developed seemingly tried-and-true patterns of thinking and reacting, crystallizing into stories about ourselves and the world, and we cling to them as our identity and home. Letting all of these constructions dissolve into the much less orderly or predictable stream of momentary reality runs completely counter to the organizing imperative of the self. There are hardly any tools in the self's repertoire, or in our collective society, for surrendering control to such an extent or for facing reality so squarely.

As we dispense with the need to make sense of *nirodha,* or to take credit for its unfolding, our usual program of trying to shape the world into a uniformly pleasant set of experiences begins to seem futile. Instead, a precious and far-reaching human faculty becomes palpable—the power to be at home in all experience, in things as they are. The central human wisdom, Patañjali teaches us, is that a pure awareness resides, impervious, at the core of each and every kind of sensation, thought, and feeling, whether we see it *(vidyā)* or not *(avidyā).* And the route to knowing this wisdom fully is yoga.

SANSKRIT PRONUNCIATION GUIDE

SANSKRIT IS THE LANGUAGE OF THE *YOGA-SŪTRA* and, for the most part, of the non-English words and expressions appearing in this book. Although Sanskrit is a direct linguistic ancestor of many English words used today, most of the important terms in yoga have no English equivalent and have therefore been included in Sanskrit alongside their translations. Furthermore, in many cases their tonal qualities are profoundly expressive of their meanings and are traditionally regarded as spiritually resonant.

Sanskrit's breadth of expression comes in part from extending yogic mindfulness to the entire vocal apparatus, multiplying the possibilities for tone production. With an alphabet of forty-nine letters, it features several different versions of familiar sounds such as those represented by *n* and *s*, each issuing from a different part of the mouth. For this reason, diacritical marks are sometimes used to indicate how and where a consonant or vowel should be sounded.

a	pronounced like "a" in *ah*
i	pronounced like "ee" in *see*
u	pronounced like "u" in *dude*
e	pronounced like "e" in *grey*
ai, ay	pronounced like "i" in *ride*
o	pronounced like "o" in *over*
au	pronounced like "ow" in *cow*
ā, ī, ū, ē, āi, āu	prolonged for two beats instead of one
h after a consonant	extra breath after the consonant (in Sanskrit there are no compound sounds like "th" in *thief* or "ph" in *phone*)
k, kh, g, gh, ṅ	*gutturals,* arising from the throat
c, ch, j, jh, ñ	*palatals,* arising from the back of the palate
o, oh, e, eh, n	*cerebrals,* with tongue touching the roof of the mouth
ṭ, ṭh, ḍ, ḍh, ṇ	*dentals,* with tongue touching the back of the teeth
p, ph, b, bh, m	*labials,* arising from the lips
c	*palatal,* pronounced like "cha" in *chop*
ṛ	*cerebral,* pronounced like rolling the "r" in *rook*
ś	*palatal,* pronounced like "sha" in *shop*
ṣ	*cerebral,* pronounced like "sha" in *gunshot*
ñ	pronounced like "ni" in *onion*
ṃ	pronounced like "n" in *uncle*
jñ	pronounced like "gn" in *igneous*
h	pronounced like "ha" in *hot*
ḥ	a soft echo of the preceding vowel

THE Yoga-Sūtra

with Commentary

1

Integration

In chapter i Patañjali defines yoga as a multifaceted method of bringing consciousness to a state of stillness. To show why this might be worthwhile, he examines what he believes to be the fundamental predicament of existence and then offers a solution. The predicament, he says, is that consciousness and the pure awareness underlying it are separate but generally feel like the same thing. Patañjali considers this the primary failure of human understanding, a defect that produces suffering with nearly every thought and action.

The solution, he asserts, is to let consciousness settle *(nirodha)* to the point where it can reflect awareness back to itself. Ordinarily consciousness is not reflective but rather a whirl of thoughts, sensations, and feelings turning in one direction, then another. When it is utterly motionless, though, consciousness becomes jewel-like, reflective enough to help awareness overcome this case of mistaken identity and recognize its true nature. This, and not our compulsive quest for gratification from external experience, is the source of the most profound happiness and wisdom.

To illustrate his worldview, or *darśana,* Patañjali introduces several key concepts, many no doubt familiar to the practitioners of his day. These include a classification of the five general patterns of consciousness *(citta-vṛtti);* the interdependent polarities of the stilling process, practice *(abhyāsa)* and nonreaction *(vairāgya);* a description of *īśvara,* the divine exemplar of pure awareness; strategies for calming and focusing the bodymind; the jewel-like reflectivity of coalescence *(samāpatti);* and the different stages of integration *(samādhi),* the threshold of realization.

1 Now, the teachings of yoga.

2 Yoga is to still the patterning of consciousness.

3 Then pure awareness can abide in its very nature.

4 Otherwise awareness takes itself to be the patterns of consciousness.

As surely as human beings are endowed with native faculties of speech, logic, and movement, so too do we possess a bottomless well of inner silence and stillness. All branches of the yoga tradition radiate from a tree whose meditative roots drank in that well for thousands of years before being mapped by Patañjali. In accordance with the ancient teachings, the *Yoga-Sūtra* locates complete realization and freedom from suffering in the bodymind's natural potential to become placid and steadily aware in the present moment.

The yoga of Patañjali is more a program for developing this capacity than it is a state to be reached. As he makes clear in chapter 2, yoga is a set of practices that "yoke" one's every aspect to the central purpose of nature—to know itself as it is. Although the word *yoga* literally means both "yoking" and "union," the idea of "yoga as union"—described in the *Bhagavad-Gītā* and certain of the Upaniṣads as the realization of unity between *ātman* (spirit) and *brahman* (universal matrix)—appears nowhere in the *Yoga-Sūtra.* Instead, Patañjali describes yoga as a system of self-refinement through which consciousness, experienced as mind and body, can come to recognize itself as a material entity, observed by an immaterial pure awareness but not aware itself.

Pure awareness, he insists, is actually not a part of ever changing nature; instead, it is immaterial, unchanging, incorruptible *seeing itself* and merely observes nature operating before it. By "seeing itself," Patañjali doesn't mean just the awareness that underlies our sense of vision but instead the omnipresent knowing before which all five senses and also the mind present themselves. Pure awareness is the knower of all sights, sounds, smells, tastes, contacts, and thoughts, yet is not *of* them.

Consciousness *(citta),* on the other hand, is the stuff they are made of. Like a television picture, consciousness arises from nature both subtle and gross. It is dependent on the conditions that created and maintain it, and utterly unable to observe itself. However, under ordinary circumstances we can't see this, instead experiencing consciousness as our self, alive and aware in the world.

Patañjali states from the outset that pure awareness is overshadowed by the modulations of consciousness, which is continually transformed from one pattern of thought to another and rarely sits still for long. This characteristic of consciousness requires deliberate, consistent, and intensive inner work, or yoking, if one is to awaken from its automaticity and see through its incessant, limiting definitions of reality.

Nature overshadows pure awareness, Patañjali explains below, because its product, consciousness, is a powerful entity that, in its usual state of commotion, obscures its actual relationship to pure awareness. Therefore, under ordinary conditions the experience of consciousness unfolds without any sense of its true purpose, which at bottom is to serve awareness. As Patañjali makes clear, though, if the agitated patterning of consciousness can be settled down, or yoked, awareness is no longer overwhelmed by the movements of nature, and this ignorance will be eradicated.

5 There are five types of patterns, including both hurtful and benign.

6 They are right perception, misperception, conceptualization, deep sleep, and remembering.

7 Right perception arises from direct observation, inference, or the words of others.

8 Misperception is false knowledge, not based on what actually is.

9 Conceptualization is based on linguistic knowledge, not contact with real things.

10 Deep sleep is a pattern grounded in the perception that nothing exists.

11 Remembering is the retention of experiences.

According to Patañjali, consciousness crystallizes the chaotic stream of perceptual events into five basic representational patterns, or *citta-vṛtti*. These arise successively, endowing our perceptual life with a feeling of continuity. Although a pattern seems to belong to a seamlessly enduring "reality" that is happening to "me," both the "reality" and the sense of "I" are actually artifacts of consciousness. *Vṛtti* literally means "turning," and the particular way that the patterns of consciousness make reality feel—namely, a field of objects observed by a subject—is imparted by their motion. This is not unlike the water in waves, which turn the surface opaque and nonreflective. When our experience is shaped by this motion, our view of things is incomplete and we suffer. When our *citta-vṛtti* turns us toward stillness, however, consciousness begins to feel more transparent and mirrorlike, providing a less distorted view.

Patañjali's universe is not relative. Some perceptions are true and others are not. We can know truth by perceiving it directly, by inferring it, or by hearing it from others. We can also misperceive, misinfer, or receive incorrect information. In either case, once we begin to imagine what our words evoke, we have subtly turned to a new pattern of thought, conceptualization, that lies at a further remove from reality than inference or testimony.

These classifications may seem strange, considering that our concepts are no more than ways to organize, remember, and clarify the truths we think we have perceived. But to Patañjali, concepts are clearly not the same thing as truth. Later, in 1.48, he shows that consciousness arrives at the highest possible level of true perception only when it moves beyond thought altogether.

It may also seem odd that Patañjali regards sleep as a pattern of consciousness. After all, deep sleep, at least, feels like unconsciousness. Imagine, though, that from the perspective of omnipresent pure awareness, or *puruṣa,* sleep is just another set of forms appearing on the screen of consciousness—in this case, dark and silent.

The last example illustrates how differently yoga defines consciousness and awareness. With consciousness *(citta),* various conditions give rise to different patterns *(vṛtti).* In the case of sleep, the patterns happen to feel like nothing at all. But no matter how patterns feel, or how they might come and go, awareness *(puruṣa)* is always behind them, unchanging and unfelt.

12 Both practice and nonreaction are required to still the patterning of consciousness.

13 Practice is the sustained effort to rest in that stillness.

14 This practice becomes firmly rooted when it is cultivated skillfully and continuously for a long time.

15 As for nonreaction, one can recognize that it has been fully achieved when no attachment arises in regard to anything at all, whether perceived directly or learned.

16 When the ultimate level of nonreaction has been reached, pure awareness can clearly see itself as independent from the fundamental qualities of nature.

Patañjali now defines the two polarities of yogic will that create the potential for realization. Practice, or *abhyāsa,* is the will to repeatedly align and realign attention to the present moment, the only place where the singular process of yoking consciousness into profound stillness can be enacted. Sustained effort is required because the forces of distraction are strong and unrelenting. Furthermore, in the first phase of stillness, they tend to increase the longer one remains immobile, as body sensations build and the impulses to move or think about what's happening intensify. At this point *abhyāsa* is easily misperceived as a struggle against discomfort and restlessness. Soon, though, one begins to regard the very sensations of discomfort and restlessness as indivisible from everything else that can be felt, and they cease to be a problem. For this reason, one must persist in returning to the here and now, holding on to the possibility of calm and lucidity, even in those moments and places where the bodymind feels under siege.

A special type of effort is cultivated and driven by *abhyāsa,* in which we practice to return to a point of focus without exertion. Instead, we come to relax the grip of wanting, aversion, or clinging to self that would pull attention away in the first place and also tend to generate subliminal bodymind tension. Thus the effort from *abhyāsa* is not overt in the same way as conventional physical or mental effort. These inevitably reinforce one's sense of self and cause suffering, as Patañjali discusses in chapter 2. That is, the more force we use, the more it feels like *we* are doing something. As insight deepens, awareness recognizes that all effort is fraught with conditioning of its own and therefore sows the seeds of future suffering in consciousness. At the final stages of stilling, all action ceases. So *abhyāsa* might better be described as "subtle effort," focused on the cultivation of effortlessness.

The will to observe experience without reaction *(vairāgya)* is the potential that brings about effortlessness. *Vairāgya* literally means "not getting stirred up" and refers to the relationship that arises in the instant one perceives something. Most perceptions pluck the strings of our attachment to various likes, dislikes, or ideals. This sets off some type of mental or physical action, which may in turn create suffering (Patañjali discusses this more beginning at 2.3). *Vairāgya* is the willingness to let a phenomenon arise without reacting to it. In other words, one can allow any feature of consciousness—a thought, feeling, or sensation—to play itself out in front of awareness without adding to its motion in any way. This subtracts more and more of the confusion from our experience, leading to profound stillness and clarity.

Thus *vairāgya* reveals the newness and originality of the unfolding moment. As we let go of reacting in conditioned ways, we are jettisoning the learned patterns we have developed in the past to relate to every aspect of experience. To let go of these is to enter into a spontaneous and unpredictable present, unmodulated by wanting, aversion, or other forms of self-centeredness. Indeed, what gets "stirred up" in reaction always has to do with *me.* The sense of "I" is largely composed of reaction, being an encyclopedic anthology of likes and dislikes, and it infiltrates even our most altruistic thoughts and deeds.

Every time we soften to an experience that would otherwise incite us to react, we break our habit of setting our personal consciousness apart from nature. As *vairāgya* extends to our most intimate, subtle, or internal reactions, consciousness begins to reflect the fact that our self—including our likes, dislikes, and ideals—is made of the same stuff as the rest of creation. All of this stuff, including what feels like "me," is in flux and subject to cause and effect. The changing properties, or *guṇas,* of this flux are no different in consciousness than in anything else. They modulate along the same lines—*guṇa* literally means "strand"—when a feeling like happiness arises and then passes away, as, for example, when a sunset comes and goes.

Patañjali's view, or *darśana,* is similar to that of another Indian system of thought, *sāṃkhya. Sāṃkhya* identifies three principal *guṇas,* or qualities of nature, that all elements are composed of, in ever changing proportions. The first is the property of luminosity *(sattva),* which rises and falls in consciousness as it grows more or less transparent and reflective, not unlike the ebb and flow of the sunset's brilliance. The second is motion *(rajas),* the kinetic quality of all experience, underlying its impermanence and attendant pain. The third property is mass *(tamas),* which confers the properties of solidity and inertia and is therefore resistant to change. Patañjali clarifies the nature of awareness by pointing out what qualities it *doesn't* have. Unlike things, awareness is *guṇa*-free, having neither luminosity, motion, nor mass. He touches upon the *guṇas* later, in 2.15 and 2.19, then details in chapter 4 how the transformation of consciousness wrought by yoga alters their appearance before awareness, thereby bringing about freedom.

Patañjali says that nonreaction is the mastery of our tendency to react. Achieving such a degree of effortlessness requires enormous effort, as he explains below. But this is a special type of effort—to allow, to let things be—that becomes refined little by little with steady practice and eventually extinguishes itself. Again, effort may be driven chiefly at first by egoic energies like wanting, aversion, or trying to become something, but every mental or physical action brought about by these energies actually produces more suffering.

For example, as we sit in stillness—meditation—we inevitably find ourselves struggling to acquire more power over some aspect of our lives. Without necessarily knowing it, we are trying to feel happy or to conquer a physical or emotional problem or to become more attractive to others or simply to do a better job of meditating than we did last time. Each of these types of effort arises from attachment to previous thoughts or actions. Even our desire to let go of all this is mired in concepts about what letting go should feel like or what it might bring us. Nonreaction means no longer operating on the basis of any of these attachments whatsoever. As Patañjali explains, though, attachments carry over from the past even as consciousness comes to settle in the present.

17 At first the stilling process is accompanied by four kinds of cognition: analytical thinking, insight, bliss, and feeling like a self.

18 Later, after one practices steadily to bring all thought to a standstill, these four kinds of cognition fall away, leaving only a store of latent impressions in the depth memory.

19 These latent impressions incline one to be reborn after one leaves the body at death and is dissolved in nature.

The stilling process unfolds in stages. In the initial stage, four kinds of mentation—analysis, insight, bliss, and self-sense—continue to arise sporadically in the midst of deepening calm. These cognitions are not everyday thought but rather are colored by the stilling process and the direct knowledge, or *jñāna,* that it brings.

From Patañjali's perspective, any kind of volitional bodymind movement, whether mental or physical, constitutes a kind of action, or *karma.* Each action or volition leaves an impression *(saṃskāra)* in the deepest part of memory, there to lie dormant for a time and then spring forth into some new, related action. This in turn will create fresh latent impressions, in a cycle of latency and activation.

Although these four cognition types produce latent impressions, some may reinforce the yoking effort, forestalling the activation of *saṃskāras* already stored in the deepest part of memory. Through these one is, in effect, holding in mind the possibility of stopping thought altogether. Consciousness eventually stabilizes to a level of calm at which such thoughts, however skillful or wise, are no longer produced or required.

This is accomplished not by exerting the will to arrest or blockade thought—an action unlikely to succeed though certain to perpetuate suffering—but by repeatedly relaxing back to the ever present object. Concentration (*dhāraṇā,* 3.1) builds spontaneously as the yogi softens and opens to experience, not through steely attempts at mind control. Eventually the only mental forms that arise in this practice *(abhyāsa)* are entrained to the same object as the preceding ones, supplanting all other perceptions. This is absorption (*dhyāna,* 3.2, 4.6). As one continues to hold on to the possibility of the mind's falling completely still, the intervals between thoughts grow longer. In time, mental formations cease altogether for minutes or even hours at a time. At this second stage, consciousness can become so tranquil that it begins to reflect pure awareness back to itself, as Patañjali describes in 4.22.

By halting its own movement, consciousness has ceased to "seed" the memory with *saṃskāras.* From then on, nothing more will be added to the store of latent impressions that were left by earlier thoughts and actions. When any of the already-stored impressions is activated, nonreaction can limit its effects by preventing it from inciting further action and thereby perpetuating the cycle of *karma-saṃskāra-karma.*

In Patañjali's view, shared by *sāṃkhya,* once action leaves an imprint, it will eventually erupt into a new thought or action. Its latency can even survive death and the body's resorption into nature's matrix, then carry over into a future rebirth. He returns to this idea in 2.12–15 and 4.9–11.

It may seem odd that Patañjali doesn't appear to place much importance in the experiences of insight and bliss that inevitably come and go as stilling deepens. Helpful and desirable though these experiences may feel in the moment, they are nonetheless subtly egoic traceries spreading turbulence across a consciousness bound for mirrorlike placidity. They may be considered landmarks indicating progress on the path, Patañjali suggests, but should not be mistaken for its conclusion, freedom from suffering.

20 For all others, faith, energy, mindfulness, integration, and wisdom form the path to realization.

21 For those who seek liberation wholeheartedly, realization is near.

22 How near depends on whether the practice is mild, moderate, or intense.

Patañjali's view of the human predicament, in which our fundamental misunderstanding about the nature of things leads to pervasive suffering, is actually optimistic. All one has to do in order to eradicate suffering, he promises, is completely give oneself over to the process of yogic realization. He also explains later (2.18, 2.21, 4.24) that the quest for liberation is entirely natural—nature, in its form as consciousness, exists to reflect pure awareness back to itself.

Faith receives its only mention here. Patañjali grounds faith not in any sort of dogma but rather in what one can truly know (1.7). So, as one sees interiorization and calm develop from the practice of yoga, one can begin to trust that further practice will yield deeper insight. This faith provides the energy for sustained practice, and the fruits of practice strengthen one's sense that realization is truly possible. This in turn fortifies one's mindfulness (*smṛti,* literally "remembering") and helps to bring about and ripen integration, the threshold of wisdom (1.46). This wisdom, or *prajñā*, specifically consists of the recognition that pure awareness exists apart from consciousness and the other stuff of creation. Wisdom is the last rung before full realization, when even *prajñā* drops away.

The special faith of the yogic path lies in the proximity of realization. When Patañjali says that it is near, he doesn't simply mean soon but also nearby. Just as an acorn holds the potential to become an oak tree, we already possess the capacity to awaken. According to Patañjali, the underlying purpose of all experience is to show us this. In a sense, perfect wisdom is woven into the very fabric of our ignorance and confusion. Pure awareness underlies all thought and perception right now, he insists, and one need only recognize it fully in order to be free of suffering.

In offering the path of yoga, though, he acknowledges the fact that profound inner stillness is required to stabilize oneself in clear seeing and that coming to stillness may take time and steady, systematic practice. The energy that goes into that practice determines the outcome, in Patañjali's equation, but this energy must not be confused with conventional mental or physical exertions, which tend to be kinetic *(rajas)* rather than quietly illuminating *(sattva).*

23 Realization may also come if one is oriented toward the ideal of pure awareness, *īśvara.*

24 *Īśvara* is a distinct, incorruptible form of pure awareness, utterly independent of cause and effect and lacking any store of latent impressions.

25 Its independence makes this awareness an incomparable source of omniscience.

26 Existing beyond time, *īśvara* was also the ideal of the ancients.

27 *Īśvara* is represented by a sound, *ōm*.

28 Through repetition its meaning becomes clear.

29 Then interiorization develops and obstacles fall away.

To Patañjali and the adherents of *sāṃkhya, īśvara* is a divine awareness that has nothing in common with any god in the pantheons of their contemporaries. Actually, neither yoga nor *sāṃkhya* is theistic per se. While Patañjali acknowledges that yogis may be inclined to invoke deities (2.44), he is careful to set *īśvara* apart. *Īśvara* is not a being or entity but rather a *puruṣa*. It was not created and cannot be destroyed, existing beyond time and space; nor does it create or destroy anything. Unlike the playful *īśvara* of vedanta. Patañjali's *īśvara* is not subject to cause and effect and is thus unmoved by devotional activities such as prayer or ritual. In this sense *īśvara* is different from the *puruṣa* affiliated with an individual. While that *puruṣa* is "coupled" to nature in a relationship (2.17–27) that Patañjali characterizes as chronically misperceived and therefore the primary cause of suffering, *īśvara* is not coupled in any way to unfolding creation.

Īśvara, therefore, is neither god nor *puruṣa* in the usual sense but rather a divine mirror toward which people throughout the ages might turn to catch a glimpse of their own true nature and its possibility of complete freedom from prakrtic entrapment. There is no actual access to *īśvara* itself, even at the point of realization; repeating the vibratory syllable *ōm* to invoke *īśvara* initiates the yogic process, eventually bringing about a nonconceptual recognition, or *jñāna,* of one's own *puruṣa*. Indeed, the phrase Patañjali uses, *īśvara-praṇidhāna,* means "aligning oneself with *īśvara*"—that is, yoking every aspect of conscious life to the perspective of pure awareness.

Interiorization is a shifting of perspective away from externality toward an interiorized point of view. In general terms, it describes the trajectory of Patañjali's eightfold yogic process, outlined in chapters 2 and 3, which crosses from orientation in the "outer world"—of people, things, and relationships—to the "inner world" of the attentional processes with which the external is seen. More specifically, interiorization is the growing sense that awareness is not seeing an object per se but instead observing a consciousness representing an object.

During the systematic practice of stilling *(nirodha),* interiorization usually begins to arise when we lock our attention on a single object or field *(dhāraṇā).* As the senses spontaneously cease to react to external stimuli, a phenomenon Patañjali calls *pratyāhāra* (2.54), consciousness begins to grow calmer and more refined in its perceptions, and capable of noticing the ordinarily invisible movements of consciousness itself. The experience is something like viewing a realistic image in a painting at the far end of a gallery. As one comes closer, the brushstrokes and the texture of the canvas become visible—eventually to the point where the image has completely deconstructed and can no longer be seen unless one elects to step back.

30 Sickness, apathy, doubt, carelessness, laziness, sexual indulgence, delusion, lack of progress, and inconstancy are all distractions that, by stirring up consciousness, act as barriers to stillness.

31 When they do, one may experience distress, depression, or the inability to maintain steadiness of posture or breathing.

32 One can subdue these distractions by working with any one of the following principles of practice.

33 Consciousness settles as one radiates friendliness, compassion, delight, and equanimity toward all things, whether pleasant or painful, good or bad.

34 Or by pausing after breath flows in or out.

35 Or by steadily observing as new sensations materialize.

36 Or when experiencing thoughts that are luminous and free of sorrow.

37 Or by focusing on things that do not inspire attachment.

38 Or by reflecting on insights culled from sleep and dreaming.

39 Or through meditative absorption in any desired object.

40 One can become fully absorbed in any object, whether vast or infinitesimal.

Patañjali lists nine types of distraction that agitate the body-mind or otherwise prevent one from being able to rest in the here and now. He also mentions three of the warning signs that indicate that a distraction has taken hold in consciousness, and offers seven ways to neutralize distraction. These seven principles of practice may derive from diverse yogic traditions already well established in Patañjali's day. As long as we settle on any one principle and stay with it, consciousness can be reoriented toward stillness.

The path of yoga, Patañjali will insist later, fulfills the primary purpose of life. Each being is representative both of all nature and of pure awareness, and its inclination toward this recognition is intrinsic. Every aspect of our being or nature, when regarded skillfully, can serve as a vehicle for the processes of interiorization and calm, and bring about realization.

In common with Buddhist tradition, Patañjali observes that the yogic process is deepened by the cultivation of friendliness, compassion, delight, and equanimity—the four "heavenly abodes," or *brāhma-vihāras*. These are radiated not just inward toward oneself and one's experience, regardless of its qualities, but also outward toward all beings. This willingness to greet all phenomena with kindliness is the basis of nonreaction (1.15).

Patañjali also makes his first mention of breath regulation, or *prāṇāyāma*. Pausing at the end of a breath phase exerts a kind of gravitational pull on consciousness, focusing it inward and away from distraction.

Another remedy for distraction is mindfulness of sensations as they arise. Ordinarily we begin to interpret and make associations at the very moment we perceive something. Patañjali here recommends fixing attention on the emergence of each successive flicker of activity *(pravṛtti)* that arises through the sensory mind *(manas)*. This is a powerful vehicle for cultivating nonreaction. The ability to rest at the razor's edge of the present, watching one phenomenon succeed another without getting caught up in chains of rumination, clarifies how the causes of suffering (2.3) breed distraction. With this clarity our relationship to our internal experience is transformed, because now we can see that our most precious thoughts and feelings are less substantial and enduring than we had realized. The steady observation of *pravṛtti* fosters interiorization, gradually revealing much more detail about momentary experience than we usually have access to, including the subtle aspects of perception *(tanmātras)*. Perhaps for this reason, *pravṛtti* have sometimes been thought of as supersensory experiences. Observing them is also calming, as the nervous system's incessant subliminal reactivity subsides.

Thoughts that are luminous and free of sorrow can take the place of distracting ones. Likewise, focusing on things that do not set off our likes and dislikes allows us to let go of the illusion that the self—the owner of those likes and dislikes—is separate from the rest of nature. All nine types of distraction are based on the illusion of a separate self.

Patañjali's final strategy for overcoming distraction is to become absorbed in any suitable object, regardless of size. As he explains at the beginning of chapter 3, fixing attention on one area *(dhāraṇā)* enables absorption *(dhyāna)*, in which the entire perceptual flow is aligned toward the object. When object is seen as indivisible from subject, integration, or *samādhi*, has arrived. These developments—*dhāraṇā, dhyāna,* and *samādhi*—arise as the relentless movements of consciousness come to a standstill.

41 As the patterning of consciousness subsides, a transparent way of seeing, called coalescence, saturates consciousness; like a jewel, it reflects equally whatever lies before it—whether subject, object, or act of perceiving.

42 So long as conceptual or linguistic knowledge pervades this transparency, it is called coalescence with thought.

43 At the next stage, called coalescence beyond thought, objects cease to be colored by memory; now formless, only their essential nature shines forth.

44 In the same way, coalesced contemplation of subtle objects is described as reflective or reflection-free.

45 Subtle objects can be traced back to their origin in undifferentiated nature.

46 These four kinds of coalesced contemplation—with thought, beyond thought, reflective, reflection-free—are called integration that bears seeds of latent impressions.

Patañjali summons the image of a jewel to evoke the transparency and mirrorlike reflectivity of coalescence *(samāpatti)*. Just as nonreaction *(vairāgya)* is the means by which bodymind stillness actually develops, coalescence is the mechanism of integration *(samādhi)*. Once consciousness has settled and become relatively motionless, its inherent—but almost always hidden—property of reflectiveness becomes apparent, as in the case of water. Now all appearances are reflected equally, and the usual distinctions between the various components of consciousness, including observer, observed, and observing itself, disappear. Subject, object, and the perceptual relationship only *feel like* individual entities—an illusion, sustained by consciousness's relentless motion, that falls away once the bodymind comes to rest.

Samāpatti is not an altered state but rather a clearer, more accurate view of experience. It means "when everything falls together" and is a completely natural way of being that arises sooner or later from the process of settling *(nirodha)*. Coalescence doesn't feel inevitable to the self, though, because the self doesn't produce it and therefore is unable either to sense it coming or to prolong it. In fact, a subtle kind of suffering can arise in the early stages of *samāpatti*, as the self finds itself alternating between a disinclination to let go of cherished distinctions and distortions, and the desire to own and control coalescence.

As Patañjali explains in 1.17 and 1.18, the stilling process develops in two stages, with the first marked by the appearance of four different types of cognition—analysis, insight, bliss, and feeling like a self. These thoughts tend to be more refined than our everyday thoughts of the same type, since they arise in relation to the calm and equanimity that are developing at that moment, and some may help maintain consciousness's orientation toward the possibility of even deeper, thought-free tranquillity.

Once this second stage arrives, the mind no longer labels an object or provides any other associations or details about it from memory. The object stands before awareness just as it is, stripped of the usual accoutrements of category and meaning with which the mind dresses up an object to set it apart from other objects: this is an apple, apples are red, I like apples.

Now Patañjali makes a further distinction, based on whether the object in awareness is gross or subtle. From the *sāṃkhya* perspective, the gross aspect of nature consists of all things that are visible, palpable, or otherwise grossly perceptible, including matter and the products of consciousness *(citta)*. The subtle elements, on the other hand, are those phenomena that are immaterial and subtly perceptible. These include the *tanmātras,* or subtle primary experiences underlying sound, form, odor, flavor, and feeling, and the movements of consciousness's three components: intelligence *(buddhi),* sensory mind *(manas),* and "I-maker," or ego-organizing principle *(ahaṃkāra)*.

When coalescence occurs in regard to subtle objects, the cognitive activity that arises in the earlier stages is subtler than the types of thought that issue from coalescence on gross objects. Patañjali calls this cognitive activity by another name, reflection, because it is less solid, more luminous and reflective, or *sattva,* in accord with the subtle objects it regards. These qualities of luminosity and reflectiveness enable awareness to know that the most personal, interior elements of being—consciousness, selfhood, and the senses—issue from the matrix of nature. As he explains in 2.6, up until now awareness couldn't perceive itself as separate from the senses. Through coalescence, this confusion can begin to be dissolved.

Lest there be any semantic misunderstanding, note that Patañjali's term here, *reflection (vicāra),* is a type of cognition, as when we reflect on experience. This is not to be confused with his image of coalescence *(samāpatti)* as being a set of states in which consciousness becomes as reflective as a jewel. In fact, only when all waves of cognition—including "reflections"—have subsided can the surface of consciousness truly become a mirror.

Together, yogic effort and effortlessness guide the bodymind as it gravitates steadily toward integration, or *samādhi.* Now that the stuff of self is no longer seen as other than the rest of creation, consciousness ceases to struggle against itself and can relax its incessant restlessness. Subject and object are no longer experienced as separate things. Put another way, as consciousness interiorizes and settles, nature appears more and more inclusive, to the point where one realizes that the self who experiences belongs to the same domain as the experience. Abiding in that realization is *samādhi.*

Samādhi (literally, "putting together") is both the culminating practice of yoga (Patañjali discusses the other seven practice components in chapter 2) and its end-state. As a practice it is the integration of the entire program, and especially the more interiorized components of *concentration* and *meditative absorption,* which distill attention to its purest form. As a state, *samādhi* is the stabilization of *samāpatti,* steadying the insight that subject and object are made of the same stuff. No longer does the sense of self set one apart from the other constituents of nature *(prakṛti);* with *samādhi,* "I" and the world have been "put together." This realization is the threshold beyond which pure awareness can begin to know its true nature.

47 In the lucidity of coalesced, reflection-free contemplation, the nature of the self becomes clear.

48 The wisdom that arises in that lucidity is unerring.

49 Unlike insights acquired through inference or teachings, this wisdom has as its object the actual distinction between pure awareness and consciousness.

50 It generates latent impressions that prevent the activation of other impressions.

51 When even these cease to arise and the patterning of consciousness is completely stilled, integration bears no further seeds.

As interiorization and calm deepen, attention can become oriented entirely to subtle objects. Gradually all cognitive activity subsides. Consciousness is now becalmed, transparent, reflective in a way that is utterly nonmental. Pure awareness, or *puruṣa,* can see and abide in its own nature. Everything that overshadowed it before—consciousness, self, the senses—is now seen as separate, as part of creation, or *prakṛti,* and empty of intrinsic awareness. This is the ultimate wisdom, or *prajñā.*

Prajñā is not a product of pure awareness, insofar as awareness neither creates nor destroys, but rather of consciousness. As the now mirrorlike consciousness reflects pure awareness back to itself, *prajñā* springs forth, creating subtle ripples of its own in the form of a unique kind of latent impression, or *saṃskāra.* This new kind effectively brings any activation of the former kind to a halt, thereby stabilizing consciousness's orientation toward realization and away from suffering.

Once wisdom is internalized thus, it too falls quiet, and no more latent impressions of any sort will be produced. Patañjali describes this as the ultimate karmic effect of integration, *nirbījaḥ-samādhi,* in which no further seeds of suffering are sown. As he explains at the end of chapter 4, the perspective that arises from this will constitute the end-state of integration, *dharma-meghaḥ-samādhi,* and fulfill the most fundamental purpose of nature.

2

THE Path to Realization

HAVING EXPLORED THE ULTIMATE STATE OF TRANSCENDENCE, *samādhi,* Patañjali now turns his attention to the route by which one comes to arrive there. After identifying ignorance of one's true nature as the root cause of suffering, he explains how it colors human experience and perpetuates itself across the span of life, death, and rebirth. To illustrate this, he describes how the fundamental qualities of creation interweave to produce experience and why that experience then overshadows the pure awareness that witnesses it. Finally, Patañjali begins to lay out the eight-limbed program of *aṣṭaṅga-yoga,* charting the path that leads from external to internal and from ignorance to realization.

1 Yogic action has three components—discipline, self-study, and orientation toward the ideal of pure awareness.

2 Its purposes are to disarm the causes of suffering and achieve integration.

The path to realization, or *sādhana,* is of no use unless one travels it. Action, or *kriyā,* is required for most of us if we are to progress toward *samādhi* (see 4.1, however). Energetic effort alone is not enough—it must be in the right direction, headed toward the supreme objective. For Patañjali, discipline, or *tapas* (literally, "heat"), provides the energy; self-study *(svādhyāya)* serves as the road map; and pure awareness, as exemplified by the divine *īśvara,* is the destination. Patañjali discusses *īśvara* in 1.23–29 and comes to *tapas* and *svādhyāya* at the end of chapter 2.

3 The causes of suffering are not seeing things as they are, the sense of "I," attachment, aversion, and clinging to life.

4 Not seeing things as they are is the field where the other causes of suffering germinate, whether dormant, activated, intercepted, or weakened.

5 Lacking this wisdom, one mistakes that which is impermanent, impure, distressing, or empty of self for permanence, purity, happiness, and self.

6 The sense of "I" ascribes selfhood to pure awareness by identifying it with the senses.

7 Attachment is a residue of pleasant experience.

8 Aversion is a residue of suffering.

9 Clinging to life is instinctive and self-perpetuating, even for the wise.

Patañjali quickly moves to distinguish between skillful action, leading to realization, and everyday action, which is mired in suffering, or *duḥkha*. Suffering has one primary cause, ignorance of one's true nature, from which four secondary causes emanate. This ignorance, or *avidyā* (literally, "not seeing"), is specifically in regard to the separateness of awareness *(puruṣa)* and consciousness *(citta)*. So, although awareness and the senses are actually not the same, they always feel like one thing, namely, a conscious self.

This self appears to "own" all of one's experience. If an experience is pleasant or positive, the "owner" is conditioned to feel attraction; if unpleasant or negative, repulsion. Either way, these conditioned reactions serve to reinforce the sense of being a self, each like and dislike forming another brick in the edifice of "I."

This self-construction takes on a virtual life of its own, seeking to preserve itself at any cost. Its flavor of substantiality and permanence are characteristic of *tamas,* the inertial quality of nature, making the self resistant to the notion of change. The more we cling to "I," the more real it feels; the more real it feels, the more we cling to it.

It is important to understand how the causes of suffering differ from skillful action. Aversion, or *dveṣa,* can serve as an example. When we are harmed by another's actions, it is wise to recognize the harm, to rectify it, and to avoid future harm. Aversion, on the other hand, is not seeing *(avidyā)* the distinction between awareness and the self and thus reflexively carrying the hurt forward by becoming identified with it. It becomes a part of "me," and the one who harmed becomes "the hurter." Mired in these identities, both we and they will have a more difficult time moving forward from the painful experience. Righteousness and guilt can seem worthwhile and may certainly appear to promote personal or social goals, but they actually prolong suffering. Neither is the same thing as clear awareness, the true foundation for taking responsibility.

Each of the causes of suffering can manifest in four ways. We typically experience one when it is activated, but it may lie dormant, stored as a latent impression. It can then erupt, intercepting and obscuring a weaker one. And as Patañjali explains, the interiorization and absorption that develop through yoga practice weaken it.

10 In their subtle form, these causes of suffering are subdued by seeing where they come from.

11 In their gross form, as patterns of consciousness, they are subdued through meditative absorption.

Earlier, in 1.45, Patañjali observes that coalescence, or *samāpatti,* allows subtle objects to be traced back to their source in undifferentiated nature. He literally says that they "terminate" there. That is, when we observe them closely, we recognize their origin as formless, impermanent, and devoid of self. Once we do, they are no longer persuasive.

For example, when we sit in meditation, even after coalescence has arisen, latent impressions may continue to form from perceptual activity. Some element of the object we're observing—pain, for example—may activate a stored latent impression, causing a feeling of aversion to bubble up. In coalescence, the distinctions that we would ordinarily apply to aversion—me/it, good/bad, tolerable/intolerable—fall away. Instead the aversion itself is revealed to be mere fleeting bodymind energies without definition, dissolving back into the undifferentiated background of consciousness from which they emerged. In this way the quality of suffering, or *duḥkha,* that ordinarily accompanies the inevitable pains and accidents of being human is seen through and can be let go.

We are not usually in coalescence when causes of suffering erupt, however, permitting them to congeal into full-blown patterns of consciousness *(citta-vṛtti),* such as the perception *I can't stand this.* At those times the pattern is neutralized as soon as we become absorbed in the perception itself. Ordinarily we answer the call of aversion by fleeing from painful perceptions. This psychosomatic tendency manifests itself both internally in the individual and in our modern culture, which teems with commercial and political messages subtly promoting the view that life can and should be uninterruptedly pleasant.

Turning to the perception itself, though, and letting awareness stabilize in it, is the essence of nonreaction, or *vairāgya,* and transforms our experience of both the perception and the perceived object. As we observe them, we come to see that their contents and qualities are in flux. Our perspective has interiorized—now we know that we're observing energies in our consciousness and that enduring entities called "pain" and "mine" are representational rather than veridical. What initially felt like solid reality—"the way things really are"—now is seen as ephemeral. In other words, gross becomes subtle.

12 The causes of suffering are the root source of actions; each action deposits latent impressions deep in the mind, to be activated and experienced later in this birth or to lie hidden, awaiting a future one.

13 So long as this root source exists, its contents will ripen into a birth, a life, and experience.

14 This life will be marked by delight or anguish, in proportion to those good or bad actions that created its store of latent impressions.

15 The wise see suffering in all experience, whether from the anguish of impermanence or from latent impressions laden with suffering or from incessant conflict as the fundamental qualities of nature vie for ascendancy.

16 But suffering that has not yet arisen can be prevented.

The cycle of cause and effect that Patañjali describes is, in fact, circular: latent impressions issue forth from the network of deepest memory as thought, word, or deed. Each of these is a type of action *(karma),* and each generates an effect that is then stored in the network as a new latent impression. Thus action begets impression, which begets action. Since the vast majority of *karmas* occur through not seeing things as they are *(avidyā),* their latent impressions are therefore imbued with one of the four corollary sufferings: egoism, attachment, aversion, or clinging to life.

We are wise, he says, to realize that there is suffering everywhere, even in the experiences we enjoy and yearn for. There is no ultimate happiness to be found in external, impermanent things. For every transitory delight we can know, a painful attachment arises. Furthermore, nature's constant transformations are subliminally stressful, relentlessly challenging the self's idea of itself as an enduring entity. And at any time, latent impressions can become activated and emerge as wanting, fear, anger, or sorrow.

As before (1.21), though, Patañjali is anything but pessimistic about the predicament of omnipresent suffering. He insists that we can break its cycle of cause and effect by yoking our attention to its source: failure to see the true nature of pure awareness and its independence from the phenomenal world.

17 The preventable cause of all this suffering is the apparent indivisibility of pure awareness and what it regards.

18 What awareness regards, namely the phenomenal world, embodies the qualities of luminosity, activity, and inertia; it includes oneself, composed of both elements and the senses; and it is the ground for both sensual experience and liberation.

19 All orders of being—undifferentiated, differentiated, indistinct, distinct—are manifestations of the fundamental qualities of nature.

20 Pure awareness is just seeing itself; although pure, it usually appears to operate through the perceiving mind.

21 In essence, the phenomenal world exists to reveal this truth.

22 Once that happens, the phenomenal world no longer appears as such, though it continues to exist as a common reality for everyone else.

23 It is by virtue of the apparent indivisibility of awareness and the phenomenal world that the latter seems to possess the former's powers.

24 Not seeing things as they are is the cause of this phenomenon.

25 With realization, the appearance of indivisibility vanishes, revealing that awareness is free and untouched by phenomena.

26 The apparent indivisibility of seeing and the seen can be eradicated by cultivating uninterrupted discrimination between awareness and what it regards.

27 At the ultimate level of discrimination, wisdom extends to all seven aspects of nature.

Patañjali now elaborates on the differences between awareness and the phenomenal world. The features of the world, encompassing all of creation including consciousness, are projected by the ever changing proportions of the fundamental qualities, or *guṇas,* at varying degrees of definition and subtlety. The vastly greater part of creation is, in fact, undifferentiated energy that is invisible to the senses. The rest of nature is manifest, or differentiated, with only a small portion composing consciousness. In turn, conscious experience consists both of indistinct properties such as the sense of "I" and distinct phenomena like perception and thought. Patañjali introduces these classifications in somewhat different terms, defining objects as subtle or gross (see 1.45, commentary).

Pure awareness, on the other hand, does not correspond in any way to the categories or behaviors of nature. It never changes, nor can it be regarded as manifest or unmanifest. It is witnessing alone, devoid of content. Therefore the phenomenal world of consciousness must be the stage not only for the earthly experience of birth, life, death, and rebirth but also for realization. Recognizing this, Patañjali asserts that the primal purpose of the phenomenal world is to reflect the true nature of awareness back to itself.

As this happens, the appearance of things changes. Like so many of the transformations detailed in the *Yoga-Sūtra,* this change of appearances must be seen directly. Just as words can describe music but can't convey it, this transformation cannot be fully conceived by the mind nor rendered faithfully in words and concepts. If it could be, we might achieve realization from books alone, and nowhere does Patañjali suggest that one could. To the contrary, each new step in the yogic process involves a greater letting go of cognitive activity so that things can be known directly as they are (1.43, for example). Words deceive, persuading us that they are the very things they merely symbolize and ensnaring us in our own conditioning.

Patañjali recognizes that there can be no substitute for direct knowing; his decision to create the *Yoga-Sūtra,* however, demonstrates his belief that words can serve to reinforce direct, preconceptual insight, even regarding transcendent states of consciousness that are beyond thought. Patañjali seems to have had practicing yogis in mind when he composed the *Yoga-Sūtra,* hoping it would organize and clarify the direct knowledge they were acquiring through yoga.

It is clear to Patañjali that the world is real, not imagined, as some of his contemporaries believed. Even though its appearance changes for the enlightened, the rest of us continue to see it the way we always have—until we too have undertaken yoga to cut through *avidyā,* or the fundamental inability to see things as they are (2.4).

Patañjali attributes this inability to a curious affinity between nature *(prakṛti)* and pure awareness. Although realization reveals them to be mutually exclusive, nature and awareness maintain a relationship through consciousness that Patañjali calls indivisibility, or *saṃyoga.* In this relationship, awareness is utterly invisible, overshadowed by the vibrant representational pageant of the phenomenal world that forms in consciousness. Thus consciousness, which arises from *prakṛti,* takes itself to be the witnessing entity. But as Patañjali points out in 4.19, consciousness is nothing but display—it can't actually see itself, and its content is visible to awareness alone.

Being able to see this fact directly is the consummate yogic skill and is called discrimination, or *viveka.* The cultivation of *viveka* requires both effortful practice, or *abhyāsa,* in the form of yoking attention to the distinction between consciousness and awareness, and nonreaction—*vairāgya*—to achieve profound stillness by letting go of having to react to any of the contents of consciousness such as sensation, thought, or feeling. Only in the total absence of internal and external bodymind movement can the presence of pure awareness be discerned.

In particular, *viveka* is the grain-by-grain realization that begins to emerge from nonreaction *(vairāgya)* and interiorization. Once it is clear that one regards not an object per se but rather one's consciousness of it, the object ceases to elicit familiar patterns of reaction, weakening its "selfness" to the point where it can be seen as lacking intrinsic awareness.

Viveka slips through the cracks of thought. Like music, *viveka* can be thought or read about but is real only when known directly. It is critically important, therefore, not to try to establish *viveka* mentally. The self-sense, *asmitā,* is almost always subtly present, avoiding detection as it lays claim to experience, and it is compelled to "own" everything, even nonmental insights. But the only way that *viveka* can arise is when the commotion of thought has subsided.

In particular, when the mind considers the *idea* of discrimination, it tends to frame it as a comparison between two tangible entities, as if holding an apple in one hand and an orange in the other. *Viveka,* however, is the discrimination between utterly intangible awareness on the one hand, and all that can be felt on the other. Thus, at first *viveka* can be experienced only in regard to the tangible. Awareness itself cannot be sensed, merely recognized by default, until consciousness arrives at a stillness so transparent and mirrorlike that its properties approximate those of awareness itself. This can develop only when latent impressions are no longer being activated or produced (*nirbījaḥ-samādhi,* 1.51, 3.8).

Viveka is not an all-or-nothing phenomenon. It develops in stages, not unlike learning to read. For example, one doesn't have to be a scholar to recognize that a row of letters on a page might be meaningful. Even a young child can identify individual letters and perhaps decode a few short words. In the same way, as discrimination develops, one begins by noticing that certain thoughts, sensations, or feelings are simply what they are and lack intrinsic awareness or permanence. Meanwhile, most other thoughts, sensations, and feelings continue to feel like "me." As discrimination deepens, more and more elements of our experience can be seen as they are, and there is a growing sense that the awareness underlying all such appearances is separate from them.

Patañjali is hardly the first author to extol the principle of yogic discrimination or to describe it similarly. As early as the fourteenth century BCE, the Upaniṣadic sage Yājñavalkya negatively defined *brahman* as *neti neti*—"not-this, not-this." *Viveka* also corresponds to the recognition of emptiness, or *śūnyatā,* as described by Siddhartha Gautama, the Buddha, when thought, sensation, and feeling are likewise seen to be empty of self. To both Patañjali and the Buddha, all experience is transparently selfless and momentary.

According to the *yoga-darśana,* the constraints of matter don't apply to pure awareness. When it is no longer overshadowed by the commotions of consciousness and knows its own nature, *puruṣa* is capable of insight into every sphere of *prakṛti,* or creation. Although Patañjali doesn't specify, he may be referring to the seven aspects of *prakṛti* enumerated in *sāṃkhya.* They are intelligence *(buddhi),* ego *(ahaṃkāra),* the sensory mind *(manas),* subtle internal senses *(tanmātras),* external senses, organs of action, and the gross elements, totaling twenty-four categories altogether. In other words, *puruṣa* has the potential to see more than just *citta,* the consciousness aspect of nature consisting of intelligence, ego, and sensing mind. Patañjali has already attributed this omniscience to *īśvara* (1.25), and it is the basis for many of the extraordinary powers mentioned in chapter 3.

28 When the components of yoga are practiced, impurities dwindle; then the light of understanding can shine forth, illuminating the way to discriminative awareness.

29 The eight components of yoga are external discipline, internal discipline, posture, breath regulation, concentration, meditative absorption, and integration.

Just as the Buddha proposed the Noble Eightfold Path as the way to the end of suffering, Patañjali conceives of the yoga program as a holistic process with eight components. *Aṣṭaṅga-yoga* literally means "eight-limbed yoking," with each "limb" meant to address a different aspect or threshold of being. The external disciplines restrain one in relation to the external world, including objects and other beings, while the internal disciplines channel one's personal energies toward realization. Cultivating a steady, mindful meditative posture grounds attention in the field of body sensation, interiorizing the yogi's perspective and enabling an extraordinary degree of relaxation. Breath regulation narrows the field of observation and deepens relaxation by exposing and counteracting the tendency of breathing to unconsciously energize turbulent mental states. Abiding in the sensations of the body as it sits and breathes brings about withdrawal of the senses, with attention shifting to an interiorized perspective. Concentration yokes the perceptual flow by funneling it to a single object or field. Absorption represents a degree of immersion in that object or field such that perceptions unrelated to it cease to arise. Finally, integration is the achievement of subject-object yoking, in which consciousness and its products—sensation, thought, and feeling—are seen to be the same stuff, their unity reflected in coalescence (*samāpatti,* 1.41).

Patañjali uses the word *aṅgam,* or "limb," to describe each component. Like the limbs of an animal, the eight components of the yoga program work together in concert. Structurally, *aṣṭaṅga-yoga* addresses eight strata of personhood, moving from an externalized to an internalized perspective. In this sense, one's path can be conceived as a journey inward—a traversal of all the layers of being, as one turns step by step away from identification with the phenomenal world of the self and objects and toward the central fact of pure awareness. At the same time, all the frontiers of being are interconnected, with the work at each supporting the work at the others. In that sense, *aṣṭaṅga-yoga* must cultivate all eight aspects simultaneously.

Thus, while Patañjali's yogic program can correctly be thought of as a progression from limb to limb, each limb develops in parallel with the others. For example, posture, breath regulation, concentration, and absorption are mutually supportive. In the meditative posture (*āsana,* 2.46), a level of steadiness and ease commensurate with realization can come about only through effortlessness, both postural and respiratory (*prāṇāyāma,* 2.49). Effortlessness can be achieved only by concentrating attention (*dhāraṇā,* 3.1) on the sensations of sitting and breathing and becoming utterly absorbed in them (*dhyāna,* 3.2) to the point of coalescence (*samāpatti,* 1.41). Then, Patañjali says, one is no longer disturbed by dualities like self/other or pleasure/pain.

Furthermore, the limbs are interactive and dynamic. As concentration deepens, it is inevitably jarred at some point by the eruption of a latent impression *(saṃskāra),* emerging as thought or action. When this is noticed, one may well reestablish concentration by briefly returning to the sensations of body and breath *(āsana, prāṇāyāma)* and watching them settle. Each phase of these back-and-forth movements may last for a fraction of a second or for minutes at a time, depending on the depth and subtlety of the practice at that moment.

It is often assumed that by *posture (āsana)* and *breath regulation (prāṇāyāma)* Patañjali meant the movements and breathing exercises of hatha yoga, widely practiced today. From this one could infer that he considered their mastery a prerequisite for integration. However, as mentioned at the outset, most hatha yoga was probably not devised until the ninth or tenth century, many centuries after the composition of the *Yoga-Sūtra,* and was almost certainly unknown to Patañjali. His modes of *āsana* and *prāṇāyāma* were far simpler, being the physical and respiratory thresholds of the yoking process, coterminous with the other six levels, their sole purpose being to serve as vehicles for interiorization and calm.

30 The five external disciplines are not harming, truthfulness, not stealing, celibacy, and not being acquisitive.

31 These universals, transcending birth, place, era, or circumstance, constitute the great vow of yoga.

32 The five internal disciplines are bodily purification, contentment, intense discipline, self-study, and dedication to the ideal of yoga.

33 Unwholesome thoughts can be neutralized by cultivating wholesome ones.

34 We ourselves may act upon unwholesome thoughts, such as wanting to harm someone, or we may cause or condone them in others; unwholesome thoughts may arise from greed, anger, or delusion; they may be mild, moderate, or extreme; but they never cease to ripen into ignorance and suffering. This is why one must cultivate wholesome thoughts.

The first component "limbs" of yoga are the external disciplines *(yamas)* and internal disciplines *(niyamas),* each numbering five. All are universal, transcending gender, age, status, or other temporal considerations.

The external disciplines, or *yamas,* are the way we yoke ourselves in relation to the world. This includes not only objects but also beings. Thus, the *yamas* guide our actions toward the benefit of all life. However, the "great vow" is not so much altruistic as practical, as Patañjali explains below, for the *yamas* benefit the individual at least as much as society, with each of its aspects bringing us around toward equanimity and insight by eliminating a set of distractions.

When we choose to follow the *yamas,* we are in effect repudiating the natural human wish, seen from infancy, for the immediate gratification of all our desires through external things. Although we learn throughout childhood to check our impulses in accordance with society's codes of behavior, every culture condones some form of violence, deception, appropriation, hedonism, and acquisitiveness. Taking the "great vow" of the *yamas* sets one apart from the rest, therefore, in allegiance to a higher standard.

The inner life of every human being is visited by unwhole-

ˏme thoughts of all sorts. Patañjali doesn't fault anyone for this, regarding it not as sin but as a natural state of affairs arising from the laws of cause and effect. He does insist, though, that only we have the power to neutralize unwholesome thoughts by cultivating the wholesome in our lives. If we fail to do this, our unwholesome thoughts are bound to manifest in some way and contribute to the cycle of suffering.

For this reason, the *yamas* must not be thought of as moral commandments but as skillful ways to relate to the world without adding to its suffering or ours.

35 Being firmly grounded in nonviolence creates an atmosphere in which others can let go of their hostility.

36 For those grounded in truthfulness, every action and its consequences are imbued with truth.

37 For those who have no inclination to steal, the truly precious is at hand.

38 The chaste acquire vitality.

39 Freedom from wanting unlocks the real purpose of existence.

A commitment to nonharming, or *ahimsā,* brings about peace in our internal environment as we become more sensitive to the ways we do subtle violence with our minds and bodies. *Ahimsā* also generates a powerful external effect, making it safe for all around us to put down their weapons and defenses. Likewise, one's truthfulness toward self and others *(satya)* not only ennobles one's personal actions but also removes the pressure to deceive that those around us may feel.

When we abandon the desire to take somebody else's belongings *(asteya),* we benefit as much as they and perhaps more. While they may remain identified and attached to their possessions, with the suffering this entails, we realize that the truly precious is all around us and can relax in the world as it is. This is the basis for the internal discipline of *santoṣa,* or "contentment."

Whatever the means of acquisition, being acquisitive is based on the deeply internalized belief that things can make us happy. Freedom from the compulsion to have *(aparigrahā)* allows us instead to seek the true source of happiness, which is wisdom, or *prajñā.*

Finally, to behave impeccably *(brahmacarya)* in all realms of conduct, including sexuality, reverses the enormous drain of psychophysical energy that takes place subliminally as our attachments impel us to misuse ourselves and others. Patañjali points out in 1.20 that energy is an essential on the path to realization. And in Patañjali's view, the costs of misconduct are inconceivable, as each digression sows a latent impression, or *saṃskāra,* eventually to germinate into more ignorant actions and resultant *saṃskāras,* in a perpetual cycle of suffering.

Patañjali now turns to the internal disciplines, or *niyamas,* each of which yokes an aspect of one's personal sphere to the process of realization.

40 With bodily purification, one's body ceases to be compelling, likewise contact with others.

41 Purification also brings about clarity, happiness, concentration, mastery of the senses, and capacity for self-awareness.

42 Contentment brings unsurpassed joy.

43 As intense discipline burns up impurities, the body and its senses become supremely refined.

44 Self-study deepens communion with one's personal deity.

45 Through orientation toward the ideal of pure awareness, one can achieve integration.

Purification, or *śauca,* extends both to the corporeal sphere of proper diet and cleanliness, on the one hand, and to mental purity cultivated by replacing the unwholesome with the wholesome. As *śauca* takes place, our relationship to the body, whether our own or another's, loses the urgency that characterizes attachment. This is an important aspect of yoking, as dwindling attachment enables expanding concentration and tranquillity.

Contentment—*santoṣa*—brings joy, not only in its momentary experience of security, but also because letting go of our attachment to externals as the source of happiness allows us to abide in the here and now.

Intensity, or *tapas* (literally, "heat"), means both austerity and zealous commitment. Although some ancient schools of yoga advocated mortifications such as fasting, there is no indication that Patañjali means anything more than the rigors pursuant to prolonged bodymind stillness. Like purification *(śauca), tapas* actualizes our commitment to know freedom by disentangling us from our attachments, snipping their tendrils one by one. Every time a distracting impulse is noted but not obeyed, the bodymind sees through and beyond it, gaining energy and inching closer to discriminating awareness.

Self-study *(svādhyāya)* refers not only to the regular, independent study and recitation of wisdom teachings but also more broadly to the way one applies them to one's own life. It is not enough simply to arrive at an intellectual, conceptual grasp of the ideas associated with tradition. One must "walk the talk" by actually taking action. Patañjali advocates attempting to follow the guidance of those who have already awakened more fully, then evaluating whether one is making progress (1.30) and acting accordingly.

Īśvara-praṇidhāna, dedicating oneself to the ideal of pure awareness, has little to do with the emotion of devotion. Rather, *praṇidhānā* (literally, "application," "alignment") is the orientation one takes as every thought, word, or deed comes to serve the goal of knowing pure awareness, or *puruṣa. Īśvara* is the landmark that points us to wisdom *(prajñā),* namely, knowledge of the existence of our own individual *puruṣa,* accessed by stilling the bodymind (1.23–29). As we sit in stillness, *praṇidhāna* is a surrender that we can make in every moment—to let nature *(prakṛti)* unfold exactly as it will, without our attachment or aversion—thereby entering the perspective of pure awareness. *Īśvara-praṇidhāna* provides the point of focus to which the yogi continually returns in the course of practice *(abhyāsa)* and the inspiration to cultivate nonreaction (*vairāgya,* 1.12–16). Finally, just as one conceives of *īśvara* as being utterly independent of nature *(prakṛti),* one comes to see the "aloneness" (*kaivalya,* 2.25) of one's own awareness *(puruṣa).*

These last three *niyamas*—intensity, self-study, and orientation toward pure awareness—constitute yogic action, or *kriyā-yoga.* The path to freedom, Patañjali insists, is a path of action and requires these three disciplines if realization is to be achieved.

46 The postures of meditation should embody steadiness and ease.

47 This occurs as all effort relaxes and coalescence arises, revealing that the body and the infinite universe are indivisible.

48 Then one is no longer disturbed by the play of opposites.

Posture, or *āsana,* is the bodily aspect of Patañjali's holistic system. Here the term refers only to those postures suitable for prolonged immobility. Strenuous, asymmetrical, intense, or ungrounded attitudes of the body would be unsuitable, since they tend to agitate the mind and cause fatigue. *Āsana* traditionally refers as well to a seat or cushion used to support the body. For most body types, a level of steadiness and ease commensurate with *samādhi* is hard to attain without such support. Even Siddhartha Gautama, a seasoned and highly accomplished yogi, bundled grasses into a comfortable and supportive cushion before sitting down to the contemplation that led to his awakening, some six or seven centuries before Patañjali.

If it is to be a limb of Patañjali's yoga, *āsana* must embody steadiness *(sthira)* and ease *(sukha)* not only in an active, external sense, as in selecting a posture and support best suited to profound stillness, but also in an interiorized, receptive way. Moment by moment we must allow our awareness of embodiment to deepen, even as each new wave of sensation buffets our attention and threatens to unmoor it from its fixation in the present.

Patañjali identifies two factors that bring *sthira-sukha* about. The first is relaxation of even the subtlest bodily efforts, almost all of which arise subliminally from suffering of one cause or another, and which promote instability. *Āsana* is a window that opens onto some of our deepest personal conditioning and the suffering it generates. In order to relax into things as they actually are, one must surrender every last drop of the internalized desire to feel good. That desire is shaped by our most cherished ideas about what constitutes good and bad, as well as by ingrained, organic perceptions of pleasure, pain, and neutrality. Both these strata are conditioned, one by prior actions and reactions, the other by the forces that combined to produce the human organism. Relaxing effort means letting go of limiting internal definitions. Simply put, in *āsana* one must do less to be more.

The second factor is the arising of coalescence (*samāpatti,* 1.41), which dissolves the ongoing stresses of wanting, aversion, egoism, and clinging to life by stripping them of their seeming substantiality. As effort descends to effortlessness, one can see the relationship between the body and the rest of consciousness more clearly. When we sit, many of the body's micromovements are just the outward manifestation of our reactivity, and the deepening physical stillness of *āsana* an embodiment of the placidity on consciousness's surface. As it calms, the surface of consciousness becomes mirrorlike, and all things—subject, object, and perceiving itself—are equally reflected in *samāpatti*. No essential difference can now be detected between pain and pleasure, internal and external, self and other, or other dualities. Likewise, the body and the external world, which usually feel like different things owing to the way the self-sense sets the body apart from the rest of the universe, are seen as appearances arising from the same phenomenal stuff. In short, it is *samāpatti* that begins to deprive the causes of suffering of the distinctions they need to exert their illusory power (2.10, 2.11), culminating in realization.

Long periods of immobility are generally required for these

factors—relaxation of psychosomatic effort and coalescence in *samāpatti*—to access and stabilize the subtlest parts of ourselves. As sensations, thoughts, and feelings evolve over minutes or hours of sitting in stillness, one cannot help but encounter unexpected new levels of intensity or restlessness. So as not to be overwhelmed by aversion or doubt, one must continually exert *abhyāsa,* the subtle effort of returning and rereturning to relaxation and coalescence. Our habit in everyday life is to shift our weight, scratch, intellectualize, or otherwise respond to unwelcome internal experiences with some sort of evasive action, usually subliminal. *Abhyāsa* here means holding on to the possibility that *this can be known without suffering*—whatever "this" happens to be in the moment. In other words, it takes a special kind of effort to achieve effortlessness.

As stilling deepens, one might question whether it is ever skillful to make adjustments to the body. To truly let go of effort, it is helpful to respond occasionally to the inevitable shifts that occur as the neuromuscular system loosens its grip on the skeleton and respiratory system. At these times, gently "stacking" the bones more vertically will actually allow effortlessness to deepen. One must, however, distinguish this from compulsive squirming and fidgeting, our habitual maneuvers to avoid suffering, or *duḥkha.*

Effortlessness instills a unique sense of freedom. As we relax, awareness begins to differentiate between the willed contractions of wanting or aversion, on the one hand, and the spontaneous, unwilled movements of energy that form the backdrop of being. Most of our active movements are learned, conditioned behaviors along well-worn neuromuscular routes, adapted for the specific purpose of grasping at the pleasant or pushing away the unpleasant. Stillness is a reflection of our growing openness to the unpredictable unfolding of the world as it is, a freedom from the constant effort to bend things to our liking, to make them conform to our conditioned notions of good and bad.

This can extend far beyond the sitting cushion. Our growing familiarity with subtle internal experiences helps us to recognize the ways our bodymind contracts in the presence of hurt, delay, desire, and other features of daily life. We begin to catch ourselves earlier in the process of tightening, viselike, around difficulty, disagreement, or frustration. We can then relax, noting how this embodies the intention to know the moment more clearly and openly. Nor is it ever wrong to do so, we begin to sense. Loosening the valves seems always to allow things to resolve and wisdom to enter. This imparts both the freedom to act and the freedom not to have to.

49 With effort relaxing, the flow of inhalation and exhalation can be brought to a standstill; this is called breath regulation.

50 As the movement patterns of each breath—inhalation, exhalation, lull—are observed as to duration, number, and area of focus, breath becomes spacious and subtle.

51 As realization dawns, the distinction between breathing in and out falls away.

52 Then the veil lifts from the mind's luminosity.

53 And the mind is now fit for concentration.

The respiratory aspect of yoking is called breath regulation, or *prāṇāyāma.* Like *āsana,* however, it arises from less, not more, physical effort. By *prāṇāyāma* Patañjali probably means something much simpler than the complex, occasionally strenuous patterns of later tantric practices. In light of these, *prāṇāyāma* (literally, "breath energy" plus "discipline, restraint") is generally regarded today as a set of practices in which one consciously directs the breath and its energies in deliberate patterns. Patañjali's emphasis, however, is different: he describes instead the process by which sustained observation of the breath without deliberation brings about natural and spontaneous changes in its qualities, enabling the deepest levels of focus and bodymind stilling, or *nirodha.*

Patañjali has pointed out that action is all too often just manifest wanting or aversion and therefore sows the seeds of future suffering (2.12–14). So it is with the breath energies, whose unbridled movements seem not only to run at a pace set by the prevailing internal state but to nourish and reinforce it. Breath energy is bridled, or "regulated," not by any attempt to impose a pattern on it, but instead by a steady observation of its qualities, which Patañjali enumerates. Whichever aspect of the breath one observes—its length, quantity, or region of activity—the effect is to make the unconscious conscious. Its rhythms no longer dictated by internal commotion, the observed breath begins to soften and spread out in each of its phases. Intervals may spontaneously occur in which the breath experiences a lull between phases. These can be gently guided, as well; although Patañjali never gets into specifics, he notes that letting the breath pause after inhalation or exhalation facilitates the settling of consciousness (1.34). Even so, steady observation alone is enough to bring about unforced changes in the breath's shape and texture. Indeed, no form of conscious, deliberate effort can make the breath as soft and unhurried as it becomes spontaneously through sustained mindfulness. And as respiration grows inconceivably spacious and subtle, it ceases to be a suitable environment for agitated mental states.

In the first, unstable appearances of *samāpatti,* one can feel how any perturbation of the breath goes hand in hand with the momentary disruption of coalescence. These perturbations usually arise from the activation of a latent impression, or *saṃskāra,* erupting into some sort of distracting bodymind state. Although it is an effect rather than the cause of this state, the breath's agitation often creates or activates other *saṃskāras,* initiating a chain of rumination and bodily disturbance. One can see how any attempt to suppress the breath might perpetuate this cycle.

Patañjali's *prāṇāyāma* brings the cycle to a halt. Absorption in the breath flow, as toward any other object, moves consciousness in the direction of interiorization and calm. Increasing stillness brings about discernment of the subtle aspects of breath—its subtle internal feelings, or *tanmātras*—and eventually coalescence. Now the play of opposites, experienced as inhalation, exhalation, and lull, equalizes, just as sustained observation of the sitting experience in *āsana* brought about coalescence and erased the distinctions between individual and universal. As coalescence stabilizes in realization—the "fourth state," *caturtha,* in addition to waking, sleeping, and dreaming—the phases of breath may disappear. Indeed, for the yogi in *samādhi,* respiratory movements can appear to cease altogether for minutes at a time.

Although such a feat may seem magical, its purpose is liberatory. When utterly undisturbed by breath and body motions, the surface of consciousness can become reflective enough to show pure awareness to itself and clarify the true nature of being. From the yoga and *sāṃkhya* perspectives, the ability of consciousness to manifest transparency and reflectiveness arises from the fundamental quality called *sattva,* which is present to some degree at all times but comes to predominate in consciousness only as the bodymind gravitates toward motionlessness. When it does, the most salient feature of consciousness is luminosity.

54 When consciousness interiorizes by uncoupling from external objects, the senses do likewise; this is called withdrawal of the senses.

55 Then the senses reside utterly in the service of realization.

Under ordinary circumstances, the senses serve experience rather than realization. That is, they are the medium through which the self identifies with experience and seeks happiness in the external objects that produce it, forming attachments and aversions to the objects found there. Withdrawal of the senses *(pratyāhāra)* reverses this. Now the senses no longer pull one's attention to distracting sights, sounds, smells, tastes, or contacts; it can stay with internal experience, even in regard to an external object, and begin to see it more accurately, as Patañjali explains at the beginning of chapter 3.

Pratyāhāra typically arises as one focuses on the indivisible sensation fields that were the objects in the two previous limbs of yoga, sitting *(āsana)* and breathing *(prāṇāyāma).* To maintain awareness of these fields, attention must narrow its scope from the kaleidoscopic panorama of multisensory inputs to just those impressions that evoke the felt sense of the body quietly seated in *āsana,* then in the more circumscribed field of breath energies.

With *pratyāhāra,* the yogi crosses the threshold of interiorization (1.29), beginning to regard objects not as compelling external realities so much as appearances arising internally. As external objects cease to compel, attention can focus more readily on one object or field, and vice versa. Only when external distractions have been completely transcended can concentration and absorption develop enough to reveal that one is always observing one's consciousness of an object and never the object itself. This is the basis of *viveka,* or discrimination between awareness and what it regards.

Nowhere does Patañjali deny that the senses or their objects are wonderful or gratifying—indeed, much of chapter 3 is devoted to the shamanic penetration and mastery of the phenomenal world—but he insists (2.18–21) that their primary purpose, and the source of lasting happiness, is realization. In chapters 3 and 4 he describes realization in greater detail.

3

THE Extraordinary Powers

PATAÑJALI, OR PERHAPS A LATER EDITOR, HAS called chapter 3 "The Extraordinary Powers" *(vibhūti).* Once attention is interiorized through withdrawal of the senses *(pratyāhāra),* the final three component "limbs of yoking" take one beyond ordinary capabilities. Together they compose the "perfect discipline" of consciousness, *saṃyama,* which can be used to master both internal and external phenomena. The power of primary interest to Patañjali is discriminating awareness, or *viveka,* arising from *samādhi* and leading to realization. Many other powers, extending to various aspects of human interest and activity, also accrue. This may be the larger connotation of *vibhūti,* which literally means "that which is extensive."

1 Concentration locks consciousness on a single area.

2 In meditative absorption, the entire perceptual flow is aligned with that object.

3 When only the essential nature of the object shines forth, as if formless, integration has arisen.

As withdrawal of the senses (*pratyāhāra,* 2.54) diverts attention from the gross realm of externals toward the internalized and subtle, concentration *(dhāraṇā)* can yoke its orientation to any chosen object or field. Once bodymind stillness has deepened sufficiently, Patañjali observes, an unprecedented fixity of attention becomes possible (2.53). This is because steady observation of the body sitting *(āsana)* and breathing *(prāṇāyāma)* is itself powerfully concentrative, and one of its primary effects is to reveal the stunning distractibility afflicting the usual modes of consciousness. This distractibility can't be rectified, after all, unless it is recognized. The "effortless effort" of *abhyāsa* manifests here as the effort both to focus and to return from distraction, while the will not to react *(vairāgya)* is the mechanism through which distractibility is attenuated. Concentration, a yogic action, and withdrawal of the senses, an effect, are interdependent, each arising with and supporting the other.

Likewise, *dhyāna,* or absorption, develops as all perceptual activity funnels to the chosen area. Any thought form *(pratyaya)* that now arises is in regard to the object or field, fortifying the stability of attention and revealing an unprecedented amount of detail. In the same way that the effect of sense withdrawal was created by the practice of observing the sensations of sitting and breathing, absorption is the eventual effect of locking attention securely on any object.

The final limb is integration, or *samādhi,* to which Patañjali devotes much of chapter 1. In the absence of its everyday commotion, consciousness settles to a mirrorlike reflectivity, and usually disparate entities like object, subject, and perceiving now coalesce (*samāpatti,* 1.41). The forms and distinctions that had individuated these entities fall away, leaving just their essential natures, recognized as the same stuff.

4 Concentration, absorption, and integration regarding a single object compose the perfect discipline of consciousness.

5 Once the perfect discipline of consciousness is mastered, wisdom dawns.

6 Perfect discipline is mastered in stages.

7 These three components—concentration, absorption, and integration—are more interiorized than the preceding five.

8 Even these three are external to integration that bears no seeds.

With the word *yoga,* Patañjali is describing a process of interiorization that begins with one's relation to externals, then to self, body, breath, orientation of attention, focus, absorption, and finally merger. Even though all eight limbs are interdependent and simultaneous, the thresholds to which they apply grow increasingly interiorized, with withdrawal of the senses *(pratyāhāra)* straddling external and internal, turning the corner toward the perspective of awareness. Seedless integration, or *nirbījaḥ samādhi,* is the ultimate attainment of interiorization, because no latent impressions, or *saṃskāras,* are being produced anymore, as is the case with awareness *(puruṣa).* As long as *saṃskāras* are produced, they will eventually be activated and erupt into action in the external world, perpetuating the familiar self-in-the-world perspective.

As noted above, when interiorization deepens, consciousness begins to reflect the fact that awareness is not actually regarding an object per se but rather conscious processes representing the object. It is the qualities of those internal processes—concentration, absorption, and integration—that can now be observed and cultivated, even if they are representing an external object.

Note that Patañjali, or perhaps a later editor, places these three components—concentration, meditative absorption, and integration—in chapter 3. As a whole, they represent a level of yoking attainment worthy of the name *vibhūti,* or "extraordinary powers." On the path to realization, they lie beyond the threshold, *pratyāhāra,* over which one must pass to enter the interiorized realm, and are said to actualize vast shamanic powers when focused on various external objects. Patañjali makes it clear, however, that only those powers of discrimination between pure awareness and the phenomenal world—*viveka*—should be given much attention. As concentration, meditative absorption, and integration are interdependent aspects of a single process, he calls them by a single name, the "perfect discipline" of consciousness, or *saṃyama* (literally "constraint," "cohibition").

9 The transformation toward total stillness occurs as new latent impressions fostering cessation arise to prevent the activation of distractive stored ones, and moments of stillness begin to permeate consciousness.

10 These latent impressions help consciousness flow from one tranquil moment to the next.

11 Consciousness is transformed toward integration as distractions dwindle and focus arises.

12 In other words, consciousness is transformed toward focus as continuity develops between arising and subsiding perceptions.

In chapter 1, Patañjali notes that when *samādhi* deepens to the point where thought ceases, the reflective experience of consciousness leaves latent impressions *(saṃskāras)* of its own; these prevent the activation of any new *saṃskāras* (1.50). Here he describes the actual transformation toward that *samādhi,* which takes place one moment at a time. Each new instant *(kṣaṇa)* of unfolding consciousness is oriented either toward or away from stillness. As more and more successive instants occur during which no distracting *saṃskāras* are activated, intervals of tranquillity begin to connect and flow together.

He then explains how the three components of perfect discipline, *dhāraṇā, dhyāna,* and *samādhi,* develop interdependently. As consciousness is permeated by longer and longer chains of tranquil moments, distractions fall away and one-pointedness *(ekāgratā)* comes about. One-pointedness is the channel to integration, involving both concentration *(dhāraṇā),* which locks on to a field, and absorption *(dhyāna),* as only mental formations related to the object now arise. Each freshly arising perception is of the same order as the preceding one, even when separated by moments of *saṃskāra*-free stillness.

Concentration and absorption are different aspects of the same yoking process, the former belonging more to the effortful domain of *abhyāsa,* the latter to *vairāgya* (1.12–16, 2.2, 2.3). Together they restrain the patterning of consciousness *(citta-vṛtti)* to the point where it is reflective, and subject, object, and perceiving coalesce (*samāpatti,* 1.41).

13 Consciousness evolves along the same three lines—form, time span, and condition—as the elements and the senses.

14 The substrate is unchanged, whether before, during, or after it takes a given form.

15 These transformations appear to unfold the way they do because consciousness is a succession of distinct patterns.

16 Observing these three axes of change—form, time span, and condition—with perfect discipline yields insight into the past and future.

Patañjali's view of consciousness appears to be generally consistent with the *sāṃkhya* perspective, or *darśana.* Consciousness is made of the same stuff as the rest of nature, although it derives from three principles *(tattvas)* unique in *prakṛti:* intelligence *(buddhi),* "I-maker"*(ahaṃkāra),* and the sensory mind *(manas).* Since consciousness is made of the same stuff, it changes along the same axes as everything else. To borrow an image used by the fifth-century commentator Vyāsa, all matter can be compared to clay. It may cycle through many forms—dispersed, collected, shaped and glazed, fired into a pot, broken into shards, dispersed once again. Each of these manifestations has a life span, a visible or knowable form, and a set of conditions. For example, the clay may survive in the form of a pot for twenty years, during which time it passes through conditions such as clean, dirty, new, old, scratched, and cracked before entering its new form, shards. But the sequence determines how change unfolds. If the potter drops the pot fresh out of the kiln, the clay will never change into an old pot, a dirty pot, and so forth. Throughout all these changes, though, the substrate—clay itself—is unchanging.

By asserting that things have a characteristic substrate that survives transformation, Patañjali is probably refuting the view expressed by certain of his Buddhist contemporaries that all matter is a projection of mind. While he vehemently opposes this view, asserting that matter is absolutely real, his viewpoint is actually not far from Siddhartha Gautama's. As in the case of the Buddha, Patañjali's realization includes the recognition that all appearances are compound in nature and thereby fundamentally unsatisfactory, impermanent, and impersonal.

Patañjali seems to base his theory of material transformation upon his observation of consciousness. In the latter, a pattern such as a memory may materialize owing to the activation of a latent impression, blaze across the screen before awareness, inspire the body to some action subtle or gross, then vanish, leaving a new impression. Four major forms of this phenomenon can be identified: impression, thought, action, new impression. One can also note or infer a time span for each form as the thought arose, presented itself to awareness, then passed away. Furthermore, each form will be marked by various conditions; other related factors might render the thought vivid or subdued, pleasant or unpleasant, brief or extensive. Nonetheless, in the *sāṃkhya-yoga-darśana,* all aspects of the pattern are *prakṛti* (nature).

If we were able to take microscopically detailed snapshots of the tableaux before us every second, we'd be able to notice subtle changes from picture to picture regarding the color, shadow, position, and texture of the objects before us. When awareness observes the act of seeing, it realizes that the visual field is never motionless, nor can it be. What is true of vision is also true for our other senses, including the awareness of thought. The seeming stability of experience is an illusion, as are the enduring qualities of objects. In fact, the universe is unfolding, expanding, advancing through time—not just as stars, planets, and gas clouds hurtling outward from their explosive beginnings, but also in our molecules, fibers, bodies, families, communities, and species. The universe's unfolding can even be sensed in our consciousness, whose flux is displayed before awareness moment by moment.

The particular nature of consciousness—unfolding as a succession of distinct patterns that, under ordinary circumstances, are perceived as a continuity—dictates how it must be transcended, as Patañjali describes at the end of chapters 3 and 4. It will become clear that wisdom consists in knowing the true nature of consciousness as a sequence of finite, inconceivably brief appearances that have no awareness in and of themselves. Only awareness *(puruṣa)* sees, and it sees without beginning or end.

17 Word, meaning, and perception tend to get lumped together, each confused with the others; focusing on the distinctions between them with perfect discipline yields insight into the language of all beings.

18 Directly observing latent impressions with perfect discipline yields insight into previous births.

19 Focusing with perfect discipline on the perceptions of another yields insight into that person's consciousness.

20 But it does not yield insight regarding the object of those perceptions, since the object itself is not actually present in that person's consciousness.

21 When the body's form is observed with perfect discipline, it becomes invisible: the eye is disengaged from incoming light, and the power to perceive is suspended.

22 Likewise, through perfect discipline other percepts—sound, smell, taste, touch—can be made to disappear.

Now Patañjali turns to the shamanic realm of yogic endeavor, which appears to have coexisted with the liberatory realm from earliest times. The appearance of magical powers in the *Yoga-Sūtra* is completely in keeping with religious traditions in India and elsewhere, stretching back to prehistory. More recently and locally, in the millennium preceding Patañjali, the possession of superhuman capabilities came to be considered a sine qua non of spiritual leadership, as the brahmanical priestly classes competed with a growing cadre of ascetic spiritual teachers *(śramanas)* whose appeal derived not so much from ritual or sacrifice as from meditative attainment. Thus, nearly every new teacher and program—including even the buddha-dharma—boasted or at least acknowledged a range of magical powers. The yogic stance, however, carefully enjoined by both Siddhartha Gautama and Patañjali, is that such powers, while impressive, do not conduce to liberation in and of themselves. This is the case even when they derive from specific activities that may, such as abiding in the "perfect discipline" of *saṃyama* (Patañjali) or in the heavenly abodes *(brāhma-vihāras)* of loving-kindness, compassion, altruistic joy, and equanimity (Gautama).

When the "perfect discipline" of the three final limbs—*dhāraṇā, dhyāna,* and *samādhi*—is turned inward, consciousness settles. One may also turn the corner, however, and observe external objects from the vantage point of interiorization, developing extraordinary powers *(vibhūti)* in regard to the observed object. Most of these either are deployed in the phenomenal world or unlock its secrets; few directly pertain to wisdom *(prajñā)*.

23 The effects of action may be immediate or slow in coming; observing one's actions with perfect discipline, or studying omens, yields insight into death.

24 Focusing with perfect discipline on friendliness, compassion, delight, and equanimity, one is imbued with their energies.

25 Focusing with perfect discipline on the powers of an elephant or other entities, one acquires those powers.

26 Being absorbed in the play of the mind's luminosity yields insight about the subtle, hidden, and distant.

Once again, the luminosity to which Patañjali refers here and throughout the *Yoga-Sūtra*—including aphorisms 2.18, 2.41, 2.52, 3.36, 3.44, 3.50, 3.56, 4.19—is *sattva,* one of the three fundamental qualities of nature, or *guṇas*. *Sattva* is the luminous, buoyant quality that gives consciousness the transparency and reflectivity that can be clearly recognized once consciousness settles. These, in turn, reveal pure awareness to itself.

27 Focusing with perfect discipline on the sun yields insight about the universe.

28 Focusing with perfect discipline on the moon yields insight about the stars' positions.

29 Focusing with perfect discipline on the polestar yields insight about the stars' movements.

30 Focusing with perfect discipline on the navel energy center yields insight about the organization of the body.

31 Focusing with perfect discipline on the pit of the throat eradicates hunger and thirst.

32 Focusing with perfect discipline on the "tortoise channel," one cultivates steadiness.

33 Focusing with perfect discipline on the light in the crown of the head, one acquires the perspective of the perfected ones.

34 Or, all these accomplishments may be realized in a flash of spontaneous illumination.

35 Focusing with perfect discipline on the heart, one understands the nature of consciousness.

Although ancient maps of the energy channels, or *nāḍī,* were passed down to the present day and may therefore still be consulted, any that might have shown the location of the tortoise channel, or *kurma-nāḍī,* appear to have been lost. Nonetheless, its function apparently was to provide energy to the emotional centers. Therefore, focusing on it with *saṃyama* is said to steady the bodymind, keeping it from being derailed by surges of feeling.

According to esoteric descriptions found elsewhere in the yogic literature, the *cakras,* or "wheels," are immaterial energy centers that distribute life force *(prāṇa)* via the *nāḍī* throughout the energetic body interpenetrating the physical one. Although Patañjali doesn't mention the *cakras* again, he lists powers that arise from subjecting certain of them to perfect discipline.

Note that it is by focusing on the heart and not on higher centers that one comes to grasp the nature of consciousness. The heart center is associated with the sense of touch, and focusing on it sharpens one's sense of bodily sensation. The yogas of both Patañjali and Siddhartha Gautama regard bodily sensation as a foundation of mindfulness and therefore a direct path to understanding the nature of consciousness.

36 Experience consists of perceptions in which the luminous aspect of the phenomenal world is mistaken for absolutely pure awareness. Focusing with perfect discipline on the different properties of each yields insight into the nature of pure awareness.

37 Following this insight, the senses—hearing, feeling, seeing, tasting, smelling—may suddenly be enhanced.

38 These sensory gifts may feel like attainments, but they distract one from integration.

Patañjali distinguishes once again in 3.36 between the phenomenal world—whose luminous quality, *sattva,* informs and facilitates perception—and pure awareness *(puruṣa),* which is separate from nature *(prakṛti)* and therefore devoid of its fundamental qualities of luminosity, activity, or inertia. It is easy to imagine how the phenomenal world—a welter of diverting qualities in constant flux, cobbled together by consciousness into a seamless whole through an enormous, near-constant expenditure of psychic energy—can overshadow the unchanging, immaterial *puruṣa.*

Developing the power to discriminate between *sattva* and *puruṣa* enables one to realize the powers of each more deeply. Patañjali's observation in 3.37 follows from earlier points, especially 3.26, where he notes that attunement to the sattvic aspect of experience greatly enhances one's sensitivity, revealing new insights about the subtle, hidden, or distant. He makes it clear, though, that the goal of yoga, and indeed the whole point of existence, is not to cultivate power in the phenomenal world but to end suffering by realizing the nature of pure seeing for its own sake.

39 By relaxing one's attachment to the body and becoming profoundly sensitive to its currents, consciousness can enter another's body.

40 By mastering the flow of energy in the head and neck, one can walk through water, mud, thorns, and other obstacles without touching down but rather floating over them.

41 By mastering the flow of energy through the solar plexus, one becomes radiant.

42 By focusing with perfect discipline on the way sound travels through the ether, one acquires divine hearing.

43 By focusing with perfect discipline on the body's relationship to the ether and developing coalesced contemplation on the lightness of cotton, one can travel through space.

44 When consciousness completely disengages from externals—the "great disembodiment"—then the veil lifts from the mind's luminosity.

45 By observing the aspects of matter—gross, subtle, intrinsic, relational, purposive—with perfect discipline, one masters the elements.

46 Then extraordinary faculties appear, including the power to shrink to the size of an atom, as the body attains perfection, transcending physical law.

47 This perfection includes beauty, grace, strength, and the firmness of a diamond.

48 By observing the various aspects of the sense organs—their processes of perception, intrinsic natures, identification as self, interconnectedness, purposes—with perfect discipline, one masters them.

49 Then, free from the constraints of their organs, the senses perceive with the quickness of the mind, no longer in the sway of the phenomenal world.

In 3.40 and 3.41, Patañjali refers to two of the five vital breaths, or *prāṇa-vāyus,* that energize different regions of the body. He never again refers to these concepts, suggesting that they—and probably the shamanic powers as well—weren't central to his system of yoga. Nonetheless, he carefully records a wide range of powers in chapter 3, perhaps to make the *Yoga-Sūtra* more fully inclusive of diverse ancient traditions, or out of deference to influential contemporaries.

Regarding 3.45, one might revisit the metaphor of clay. Its gross aspect includes what we can feel, see, and smell, whereas its subtle properties can be known only through *saṃyama,* or by scientific inference. Likewise, its intrinsic properties set it apart from other matter, as do the ways it relates and interacts with other elements. Finally, its purpose may be known. As before, Patañjali's ideas reflects the *sāṃkhya-darśana,* which enumerates twenty-four aspects of *prakṛti,* including the elements, the senses, and consciousness, but makes no distinction between them regarding modes of transformation. Thus one can master the sense organs, for example, with the same approach—*saṃyama*—that one used to penetrate the mysteries of clay.

As interiorization proceeds, consciousness withdraws the senses from gross external objects, turning instead to subtle internal ones. Perfect discipline *(saṃyama)* directed at the perceptual process itself means interiorizing to the point at which the subtle aspects of sensing, the *tanmātras,* become visible in consciousness. To grasp this conceptually, consider the chain of perception that occurs as we hear a sound. The object, an audible vibration in the air, reaches an organ of perception (the ear) that transduces the vibration into another medium, the sense of hearing; this surfaces as an impression in consciousness, where it is stratified and brought into coherence with all the other sense inputs by the sensory mind *(manas)* in concert with the other components of consciousness, intelligence *(buddhi)* and ego *(ahaṃkāra).* As the sensory mind collates these inputs, conditioned reactions arise in intelligence and ego that welcome certain inputs, filter others, and produce the organized mental representation we experience as the sound. As intelligence *(buddhi)* and ego *(ahaṃkāra)* color the sensory projection, the subtle internal sense *(tanmātra)* evokes the hearing experience, or soundness, of the phenomenon. *Tanmātras* are always present in the perceptual chain but ordinarily cannot be contemplated in isolation, since they fuse with the other cognitive aspects of perception. Only in the transparency of *saṃyama* can the mental overlay be seen through and the subtle essence of hearing be observed (3.3). The *tanmātra* of hearing is now "free from the constraints of its organ"—that is, the other, bodily links in the auditory sequence.

At this level of discrimination, the different flavors of subtle sensual experience arise and pass away like quicksilver, friction-free, buoyantly sattvic. They are no longer encumbered by the more external, tamasic links of the chain. This is the "great disembodiment" *(mahā-videha),* a milestone on the path of interiorization indicating that bodily attachment has receded and that luminous *sattva* now predominates in consciousness.

50 Once one just sees the distinction between pure awareness and the luminous aspect of the phenomenal world, all conditions are known and mastered.

51 When one is unattached even to this omniscience and mastery, the seeds of suffering wither and awareness knows it stands alone.

52 Even if the exalted beckon, one must avoid attachment and pride, or suffering will recur.

The quality called *sattva* accounts for the luminosity and clarity of the phenomenal world. *Sattva* is the particular quality of consciousness—and by extension *prakṛti*—that is most easily mistaken for the seeing of pure awareness *(puruṣa),* which is actually devoid of qualities. In profound stillness, with consciousness at its most reflective, discrimination begins to appear. The critical juncture is that point at which pure awareness is recognized to be different from *sattva. Sattva* comes to predominate in consciousness through the processes of interiorization and calm, as consciousness manifests a natural transparency and a reflectiveness that are hardly visible under ordinary circumstances. Now consciousness mirrors pure awareness back to itself for the first time, and discrimination *(viveka)* arises.

Any attachments that remain will set off wave-making thoughts or actions, disturbing the glassy surface of consciousness. But as long as one can maintain this critical discrimination between pure awareness and *sattva,* and not be jolted by the eruption of distracting *saṃskāras,* the liberating realization of *kaivalya,* or *puruṣa*'s separateness from *prakṛti,* can unfold.

53 Focusing with perfect discipline on the succession of moments in time yields insight born of discrimination.

54 This insight allows one to tell things apart that, through similarities of origin, feature, or position, had seemed continuous.

55 In this way discriminative insight deconstructs all of the phenomenal world's objects and conditions, setting them apart from pure awareness.

56 Once the luminosity and transparency of consciousness have become as distilled as pure awareness, they can reflect the freedom of awareness back to itself.

At the conclusion of the *Yoga-Sūtra* in chapter 4, Patañjali will elaborate on the mind-bending concepts introduced in these four final *sūtras*. In them Patañjali is describing one of the key insights of end-state *samādhi*. By remaining absorbed in the procession of momentary events, one recognizes that what had seemed a continuous flow of reality reveals itself to be a sequence of consciousness moments, each composed of irreducible perceptual phenomena, or *dharmas*. This becomes visible because perfect discipline, or *saṃyama,* seems to elongate the temporal experience. As noted in 1.41 and 3.3, the coalescence that arises in *samādhi* relaxes forms and distinctions, including temporal constraints. An indescribable wealth of detail can now be seen, as the subtle aspects of nature arise in rapid succession. One can now directly know the granular substrate of all conscious experience, each of its particulate transformations unfolding in the smallest perceptible instants of time *(kṣaṇas)*. The illusion that this stuff is seeing itself has finally been destroyed.

4

Freedom

At the end of chapter 3 Patañjali leaves us with a glimpse of freedom, or *kaivalya.* As he defines it, *kaivalya* is not a state that we achieve but rather the inherent separation that exists between *prakṛti* and *puruṣa.* Recognition of this separation is called discrimination, or *viveka,* and is accompanied by insight into the momentary transformations of the world's forms. It is this insight that defuses the dramas of consciousness, in effect freeing it from further suffering.

In chapter 4 he prepares us for a more thorough depiction, elaborating on the way forms arise in nature and continually change. He describes the latent forces that drive these transformations, both of consciousness and of its objects. He then analyzes and affirms the reality of the world, independent of the perceptions of its observers. Consciousness itself is an object, he asserts, incapable of self-regard. Once its recognition as such can be steadily maintained, reality can finally be seen as it actually is—a torrent of microphenomena utterly devoid of substantiality or permanence. The true nature of pure awareness itself is now visible, omnipresently observing the world but separate from it and not imbued with its qualities. This, Patañjali explains, fulfills the true purpose for which nature created consciousness, and marks the end of suffering.

1 The attainments brought about by integration may also arise at birth, through the use of herbs, from intonations, or through austerity.

Patañjali begins the final section of the *Yoga-Sūtra* with a surprising revelation: the extraordinary powers, or *vibhūti,* are not unique to the yogic process. That is, they may arise spontaneously from causes other than perfect discipline. He doesn't indicate, however, whether they manifest in a form suitable for the purpose of liberation.

2 Being delivered into a new form comes about when natural forces overflow.

3 The transformation into this form or that is not driven by the causes proximate to it, just oriented by them, the way a farmer diverts a stream for irrigation.

The forces that give rise to change exist before change becomes visible. Patañjali uses the example of a farmer to distinguish between the forces that create a new form and the proximate causes surrounding its emergence. The farmer doesn't generate the water or its force but merely directs it.

Another metaphor related to cultivation might make Patañjali's concept even clearer. A farmer doesn't actually create a crop such as apples; rather, they are the product of apple trees, each one the latest in a long line of predecessors. The ancestry of each apple tree stretches back to antiquity, every generation depending for its existence on a fruitful convergence of seed, sunshine, water, and nutrient soil. The farmer, as the current agent of convergence, is a proximate cause of the apple's existence, having obtained the seeds, planted them in rows of soil, irrigated and fertilized them, and finally harvested the fruit. One would even call the product "the farmer's apples." But it is primarily the seed that determines the apple's essential attributes—color, texture, taste, shape, content, life span, and potential to reproduce—even though each of these may be affected by proximate causes.

In the same way, it is the "seed" of the latent impression *(saṃskāra)* that germinates, blooming into specific thoughts, forms, and actions. The set of conditions that host this emergence will certainly influence it, like the farmer's influence on the apple crop, but its essential attributes are determined long before it becomes visible.

4 Feeling like a self is the frame that orients consciousness toward individuation.

5 A succession of consciousnesses, generating a vast array of distinctive perceptions, appears to consolidate into one individual consciousness.

Likewise, in Patañjali's view the forms of nature that we experience as our "self" are brought about by the overflowing of natural forces, in this case the activation of *saṃskāras* that, like apple seeds, determine our essential attributes. There is also an important proximate cause, called *ahaṃkāra* in the *sāṃkhya* system. *Ahaṃkāra* is the individuating principle, or "I-maker." Like the farmer, it organizes the chaotic infinitude of internal and external processes into what feels like a single person, from infant to elder. Even though a being may experience countless, often radically different modes of consciousness, each erupting from the activation of latent impressions, *ahaṃkāra* impregnates them all, regardless of their variety, with a unifying self-sense, or *asmitā*. This makes them all feel like they're "happening to me."

6 Once consciousness is fixed in meditative absorption, it no longer contributes to the store of latent impressions.

7 The actions of a realized yogi transcend good and evil, whereas the actions of others may be good or evil or both.

8 Each action comes to fruition by coloring latent impressions according to its quality—good, evil, or both.

9 Because the depth memory and its latent impressions are of a piece, their dynamic of cause and effect flows uninterruptedly across the demarcations of birth, place, and time.

10 They have always existed, because the will to exist is eternal.

11 Since its cause, effect, basis, and object are inseparable, a latent impression disappears when they do.

Absorption, or *dhyāna,* is a critical mechanism in the yoking process. Before it arises, the patterning of consciousness *(citta-vṛtti)* rolls inexorably forward, like a gargantuan juggernaut careening in one direction, then another, leaving tracks wherever it goes. In *dhyāna,* though, all perceptual activity aligns with an object, and the *citta-vṛtti* juggernaut ceases to turn this way and that, instead coming to a stop in one place. No further impressions are made in the ground other than where it now stands, leaving the rest of its surface smooth. Only then can *samādhi* develop, with the mirror of coalescence showing things as they are, devoid of the distinctions (1.43) that had left behind an unbroken trail of attachments and aversions.

Eventually, Patañjali says, actions born of ignorance and programmed for suffering cease to arise. The acts of the realized yogi cannot leave any residue. It is comforting to imagine the possibility of a being who no longer errs, but Patañjali is only speaking of those at the ultimate level of realization, *dharma-meghaḥ-samādhi* (4.29, 4.30), which is not often attained.

For the rest of us, actions do leave residues, in the form of *saṃskāras.* According to *sāṃkhya,* these accumulate in a residuum *(āśaya),* which, like the *saṃskāras,* is not part of the physical body.

Instead they are located in the subtle body *(liṅgadeha),* which survives death and rebirth. Patañjali indicates that the *saṃskāras* are driven by an irresistible animus, the will to exist, which produces the inclination to be reborn (1.19).

Each *saṃskāra* has four attributes: a cause, usually originating with one of the five causes of suffering *(kleśas);* an effect, manifested as thought or action *(karma);* a basis in consciousness *(citta);* and the support of an object *(viṣaya).* Patañjali mentions this in order to explain how *saṃskāras* are deactivated at the time of ultimate realization, which he discusses beginning with 4.29. Not only does realization eradicate the causes of suffering, as well as cause and effect, but it also represents a transformation in which the ordinary appearances of consciousness and the phenomenal object world are seen through. Since the four *saṃskāra* attributes are inseparable, the dissolution of a single one means the end of the *saṃskāra* as well.

12 The past and future are immanent in an object, existing as different sectors in the same flow of experiential forms.

13 The characteristics of these sectors, whether manifest or subtle, are imparted by the fundamental qualities of nature.

14 Their transformations tend to blur together, imbuing each new object with a quality of substantiality.

Any object or phenomenon consists of a succession of moments in which innumerable experiential forms, or *dharmas,* arise and pass away. These cannot ordinarily be perceived as such, instead running together like the frames in a motion picture. This tendency to blur together imparts an unreal sense of continuity and permanence to phenomena, an illusion that is nonetheless taken to be their actual reality. Indeed, while Patañjali's word *dharma* never means anything in the *Yoga-Sūtra* other than "irreducible constituent of experience," *dharma* is one of the most inclusive words in the Sanskrit language and commonly refers to several different orders of reality, both micro- and macroscopic. Other traditional meanings include "nature as a whole," "the lawfulness of natural processes," "teachings related to natural law," "mental state," and "the virtue that arises from living in accord with nature." It also widely refers to the Buddhist perspective *(darśana),* including practices and teachings.

In the case of a movie, the rapidity of its transformations, at twenty-four frames a second, lies beyond the range of our perceptual ability. Though we may know conceptually that the motion on the screen is illusory, we cannot distinguish a single frame, no matter how hard we try. The mind and its products are different, though. The turbulence of everyday mental patterning contributes enormously to our inability to differentiate its rapid sequence of perceptual events. As the mind settles, we can see increasingly subtle grades of transformation, eventually including those of the *guṇas* (4.33), which contribute the varying proportions of light, motion, and mass characteristic of each object or phenomenon.

Each transformation is conditioned by the reality that existed just an instant *(kṣaṇa)* earlier. In other words, the world and its objects, including consciousness, may be thought of as a lawful, orderly procession of effects arising from previous causes and generating their own, later effects. In this view, the present consists of the past and the future, which are merely different stretches of the same river. Patañjali explained in 3.16 that this truth is not merely an inference but can be known directly *(jñāna)* through perfect discipline.

15 People perceive the same object differently, as each person's perception follows a separate path from another's.

16 But the object is not dependent on either of those perceptions; if it were, what would happen to it when nobody was looking?

17 An object is known only by a consciousness it has colored; otherwise it is not known.

The world, Patañjali assures us, is real, and its objects exist independently of the observer. Like the object, the act of observing can be broken down into constituents. Every perception may traverse several of the strata that compose a human being, including sense organs *(indriya)*, sensory mind *(manas)*, intelligence *(buddhi)*, "I-maker" *(ahaṃkāra)*, and subtle sense experiences *(tanmātras)*. These constitute the "path" along which the sensing of an object travels on the way to becoming a full-fledged perception. As Patañjali pointed out in 2.27, wisdom, or *prajñā,* clarifies the actual nature of each of these strata. Even in the absence of *prajñā,* though, one can readily understand how any path through these strata cannot be the same from one person to the next. And if this sensing never reaches consciousness—namely, intelligence, I-maker, and sensing mind—it cannot be known.

18 Patterns of consciousness are always known by pure awareness, their ultimate, unchanging witness.

19 Consciousness is seen not by its own light but by awareness.

20 Furthermore, consciousness and its object cannot be perceived at once.

21 If consciousness were perceived by itself instead of by awareness, the chain of such perceptions would regress infinitely, imploding memory.

22 Once it is stilled, though, consciousness comes to resemble unchanging awareness and can reflect itself being perceived.

23 Then consciousness can be colored by both awareness and the phenomenal world, thereby fulfilling all its purposes.

Now Patañjali hones in on a key distinction between awareness and consciousness: the latter is the object of the former and cannot illuminate itself. In other words, consciousness cannot see itself, any more than a television picture can watch itself, even though it is capable of displaying a vast array of distinctive programs and settings, each offering a compelling pseudo-reality. Once the volume is turned down and the screen darkened, however, the illusion evaporates. One remembers that it was just a show appearing on a machine. Seeing our reflection in the screen, we sense ourself sitting there, breathing, watching, thinking.

To penetrate to Patañjali's view of realization, we must go beyond this metaphor. One awakens from the illusory experiences of sitting, breathing, watching, and thinking—the pageant of the phenomenal world—to the knowledge of pure awareness, standing apart from all experience. Nobody is watching. There is just watching itself—*puruṣa*.

Patañjali explains that an object becomes a percept by "coloring" consciousness. Thus, once consciousness is becalmed to the point of resembling pure awareness, *puruṣa* can sense its own presence for the first time. Consciousness is now "colored" by awareness and can represent it back to itself. In its luminosity, consciousness reveals more of the detail about itself and the transformations of its constituent stuff—insights that will ultimately unravel the bonds of the *guṇas* and their projections.

Patañjali asserts that the phenomenal world is the ground for both experience and liberation (2.18). Now that consciousness can accommodate both aspects of existence, *prakṛti* and *puruṣa,* both its purposes can be fulfilled, and freedom is at hand.

24 Even when colored by countless latent traits, consciousness, like all compound phenomena, has another purpose—to serve awareness.

25 As soon as one can distinguish between consciousness and awareness, the ongoing construction of the self ceases.

26 Consciousness, now oriented to this distinction, can gravitate toward freedom—the fully integrated knowledge that awareness is independent of nature.

27 Any gaps in discriminating awareness allow distracting thoughts to emerge from the store of latent impressions.

28 These distractions can be subdued, as the causes of suffering were, by tracing them back to their origin, or through meditative absorption.

All things are composite in nature, consisting of irreducible experiential forms (dharmas) whose transformations occur in the briefest instant *(kṣaṇa)* and are imbued with fundamental qualities *(guṇas)* in ever changing proportions. Consciousness is just such a thing, like all the other entities composing the world of things. As Patañjali describes earlier (2.18, 2.21), this phenomenal world of *prakṛti* exists and evolves in essence to reveal *puruṣa* to itself, in so doing also exposing the true nature of *prakṛti*.

At first consciousness can remain only briefly in the profound stillness necessary for mirroring. Latent impressions sown by the causes of suffering continue to erupt into thoughts or actions, stirring up consciousness and reducing its transparency and reflectivity. The causes of suffering, whether subtle or gross in nature (2.10, 2.11), can be neutralized, however, through returning to the point of focus *(abhyāsa)* and nonreaction *(vairāgya)*. Once they are neutralized, profound stillness grows increasingly stable, until one arrives at the ultimate stage of nondoing.

29 One who regards even the most exalted states disinterestedly, discriminating continuously between pure awareness and the phenomenal world, enters the final stage of integration, in which nature is seen to be a cloud of irreducible experiential forms.

30 This realization extinguishes both the causes of suffering and the cycle of cause and effect.

31 Once all the layers and imperfections concealing truth have been washed away, insight is boundless, with little left to know.

32 Then the seamless flow of reality, its transformations colored by the fundamental qualities, begins to break down, fulfilling the true mission of consciousness.

33 One can see that the flow is actually a series of discrete events, each corresponding to the merest instant of time, in which one form becomes another.

34 Freedom is at hand when the fundamental qualities of nature, each of their transformations witnessed at the moment of its inception, are recognized as irrelevant to pure awareness; it stands alone, grounded in its very nature, the power of pure seeing. That is all.

The cloud of irreducible experiential forms, *dharma-megha,* is Patañjali's description of the ultimate state of human perception. It is observing things at their most basic level, in the briefest increments of knowable time. It is reality, stripped of the drama with which the *guṇas* saturate ordinary perception. For Patañjali it is the supreme realization, not only of human yoking, but of nature's purpose—to be seen exactly as it is.

Dharma-megha can be discerned only when the surface of consciousness has been stilled of all patterning. Once it is utterly stable, it behaves like a mirror reflecting pure awareness, or *puruṣa,* back to itself. Patañjali also describes, in 4.23, how this reflection colors consciousness, enabling it to represent its own constituents more in the way of pure awareness. Thus consciousness transparently reflects the unfolding of phenomena as they are at the most granular level, unclouded by any constructive or organizing mental activity whatsoever.

Awareness *(puruṣa)* is not subject to the forces that govern matter and consciousness; it is entirely beyond cause and effect. Like *īśvara,* it also transcends time. Because consciousness belongs to the realm of the world, its contents are constrained by temporality, but the vision of pure awareness does not. Standing alone, it can see the briefest instants of transformation, while the *guṇas'* qualities are projected on the flux of consciousness stuff. This is radically different from everyday perception, whose transformations blur together to present a seamless continuity, even when consciousness is nearly motionless. Like the frames of a movie, it is this continuity on which the drama of selfhood depends. Once the continuity breaks down, the drama vanishes.

Although its surface can become placid enough to present a mirrorlike reflection back to pure awareness, consciousness is prakrtic in nature. Thus it arises in the form of perceptual elements that are in constant motion. These are called *dharmas,* the fleeting granular forms that combine to produce what seems like a unitary flow of experience. Whereas subatomic particles are the smallest physical constituents and must be inferred scientifically, a *dharma* is the briefest constituent phenomenon of consciousness that awareness can observe directly.

Under ordinary circumstances, *dharmas* appear to run together, lending a singularity and substantiality to what is actually compound and evanescent. In the final *samādhi,* though, these unimaginably brief microphenomena are seen distinctly by pure awareness. All things are recognized as compound and illusory projections of gunic luminosity, motion, and solidity, and cease to compel. It is now seen that the *dharmas* don't run together after all but flicker discretely before awareness.

Although *meghaḥ* has the specific connotation of "cloud," Patañjali appears to intend something subtler and more inclusive of *meghaḥ*'s larger meaning, "rain shower." *Dharmas* rise to the surface of consciousness—and thereby become visible to pure awareness—at different moments, the way raindrops arrive separately at the ground from above. However, because the intervals between these arrivals are so brief, they are experienced as one big thing rather than countless small ones, except at the most radical degree of bodymind stillness. In other words, though the untrained hear nothing but the continuous rush of water, the realized perceive all arrivals distinctly.

There can be no shower without a cloud, however. Once

the surface of consciousness has become a mirror and therefore reflects itself more clearly, pure awareness is able to recognize the continuous nature of consciousness's patterns *(citta-vṛtti)* as nothing more than a succession of *dharmas.* This *dharma* stream is the indivisible matrix of what can be known, the particulate stuff constituting all of consciousness's motions *(vṛtti),* and appears cloudlike to the pure awareness that has become disidentified with it.

Recalling the motion picture metaphor, if *vṛtti* can be likened to the ever changing tableaux in the movie itself—with the fundamental qualities of experience, the *guṇas,* projecting shifting proportions of light, motion, and density—the *dharmas* are the granular frames composing the continuous medium that is the film itself. Like a movie, each reality tableau appears to unfold in a seamless flow. But when we stop the projector and study that section of the filmstrip under a microscope, we see both the sequentiality of the individual frames and the contiguous granular field that is their matrix. What can no longer be readily seen is the illusion of motion *(vṛtti).* Just as the frames are individual but belong to a single filmstrip, *dharma-megha* shows pure awareness that the segregation of time into past, present, and future is a form of mental patterning superimposed on the unitary *dharma* cloud.

The movie metaphor is not completely satisfactory, however. In that segment of the filmstrip, each of the frames depicts roughly the same visual composition, with only subtle changes from frame to frame. *Dharmas*, on the other hand, correspond to sights, sounds, smells, tastes, contacts, and also mental objects like thought and emotional feeling; therefore, a single *dharma* represents only a small portion of any given tableau.

Once consciousness has become completely disidentified with awareness, the causes of suffering, five in number but all predicated on an inability to see the true nature of *prakṛti* and *puruṣa,* are abolished. Without them, no further seeds of ignorant thought or action can be sown, and those already stored vanish (4.11). These are the layers that concealed the true nature of things; once they are gone, nothing remains standing in the way of complete realization.

The *guṇas* depended for their effects on the relatively gross calibrations of everyday perception. But in the absence of any bodymind movement whatsoever, consciousness now can reflect the finest possible grade of phenomena. At this level of discrimination, the *guṇas'* contribution to the coloring of each new transformation can clearly be seen. Once seen through, the *guṇas* lose all power to compel, and become irrelevant.

Patañjali assures us that the world of objects and their qualities are real (4.15, 4.16) but cannot be perceived uniformly by different observers. Fully realized awareness regards exactly the same world as it did prior to realization, and exactly the same world that others now see. Its appearance, and the effect of its qualities, are utterly and irreversibly altered, however.

As in the case of *samāpatti, dharma-meghaḥ-samādhi* must not be conceptualized as an altered state. Though both constitute radical departures from conventional modes of experience, neither "feels" like anything other than *things as they are,* albeit in more basic, distilled forms. The contents of these states are always present, whether seen during realization or when occluded by rampant representational activity *(citta-vṛtti).* As in the buddha-dharma, which acknowledges the ever-presence of emptiness and *nirvāṇa* (Pali: *nibbāṇa*), Patañjali's reality is always a cloud of *dharmas* that are sequentially arising and vanishing at an inconceivable rate. To Patañjali the world is never otherwise; when stilling is effected, the true nature of things becomes apparent. Thus, for the yogi who practices wholeheartedly (1.21), realization is always at hand.

In the actualized state of *dharma-meghaḥ-samādhi,* consciousness no longer contributes anything at all to the pageant of phenomena. The drama inherent in birth, experience, suffering, and death is at an end, replaced by inexpressible knowledge. Awareness can now see its own reflection: unchanging, independent, utterly unaffected by the flux of phenomenal energies. This is the attainment of the yogic ideal, attributed by Patañjali to the divine awareness *īśvara* but actually, like all divinity, dwelling as the deepest human possibility in each and every one of us.

Afterword

The Yoga-Sūtra *Today*

The legacy of the *Yoga-Sūtra* is vast. Today it is possible to view Patañjali's work through many lenses. As a philosophical system, it has taken its place as the definitive statement of the *yoga-darśana,* one of six orthodox schools of Indian thought. From an historical or anthropological perspective, it is a remarkable artifact, an ancient sacred text that comprehensively expresses a system of thought and conduct reflecting the culture of an earlier time and place. Linguistically it is an inexhaustible trove, brimming with mellifluous Sanskrit euphonies and elegant phraseology, and in spite of enormous scope, a masterpiece of concision.

First and foremost, however, the *Yoga-Sūtra* continues to compel chiefly because of the way it addresses the central concerns of human existence. Although we know nothing of its author save the name Patañjali, we can be certain that he was devoted, along with countless predecessors, to the eradication of suffering. Because he believed that human suffering stems from an ingrained but reversible tendency to misconstrue reality, he undertook a painstakingly thorough analysis of how we know what we know. It is this inward journey, made accessible to all, that is so universal and inspiring, and it is Patañjali's trail that we attempt to retrace, step by step, once we've taken the *Yoga-Sūtra* to heart and made our first strides on the path to freedom.

Naturalness and simplicity are the *yoga-darśana's* great virtue. No matter what object or aspect of experience one might choose to contemplate, the observing process will gradually come to reveal the awareness underlying it. To Patañjali the supreme purpose of the phenomenal world is to evolve to the point where it can reveal the great interlocking truths: that awareness is intrinsically free and that every human being can come to know freedom. Patañjali unshackles us from the fetters of conventional effort, which largely belongs to the domain of suffering, and instead directs us to the possibility of effortlessness. The yogic processes of interiorization and calm are not as much something *we do* as they are naturally unfolding properties of being that our selves usually hold in check.

Patañjali seems to have recognized that the greatest challenge for students of the *yoga-darśana,* and therefore the great barrier to transmission, is the fact that we tend to encounter the possibility of bodymind cessation first as a concept that we hear or read about. Because of this fact, we cannot help but form ideas about what realization is and try to bring them about mentally. This cannot produce the imagined result, though, any more than one can slake a thirst by thinking about water.

Yogic practice does depend for its success, though, on the way that the yogi accepts and incorporates certain ideas *(pratyayas)* to shape behavior and experience, continually reorienting them toward realization. For example, one must develop an understanding of the yogic program itself, remembering the necessity of relaxation, focus, and persistent returning to the present. One must also hold in mind the possibility of utter mental cessation and realization, a potential one comes to detect in all experience.

An important feature of the *Yoga-Sūtra* is Patañjali's emphasis on embodiment. *Āsana* and *prāṇāyāma* are the ground of the yogic path. With the body and all its phenomena ever in view, their impermanence and lack of selfhood come into focus as stillness, or *nirodha,* develops. The futility of clinging to this corporeal life-as-a-self also becomes apparent. Indeed, the dependent, conditioned flow of cause and effect that mind labels as *the body* can only be seen as devoid of intrinsic awareness or permanence when it remains under the continuous scrutiny Patañjali recommends for yogic awakening.

This emphasis on physical sensation, also notable in the teachings of the Buddha, is not theoretical but rather a pragmatic response to experience and practice. Conceptually, Patañjali appears to share the *sāṃkhya* view that what awareness regards is a display generated by a tripartite consciousness consisting of sensing *(manas),* self-making *(ahaṃkāra),* and intelligence *(buddhi).* These three components have radically different properties: thought, emotion, and feeling like a self are all constructive in nature, arising actively as latent impressions *(saṃskāras)* erupt against a background of sensory inputs mediated by the nonconstructive *manas.* These impressions color and organize all aspects of perception, linking them in cycles of action-imprint-action that are imbued with suffering. However, when attention is yoked to the sensory field and steadily maintained there, one eventually becomes sensitive to the subtlest emergences of thought, feeling, and I-ness. Any such constructive activity begins to stand out, acquiring a transparency that allows it to be recognized for what it is: a mental product that is conditioned, impersonal, and nonmandatory.

Although the sensory domain conveyed by *manas* is nonconstructive per se, it is the field in which the most primal human urges and repulsions germinate. Hunger, thirst, fatigue, lust, and pain are all perceptions with an experiential core of sensation, seemingly swathed in selfness at inception. When the will not to react *(vairāgya)* is applied to the sensory field from moment to moment, though, the self's possessive grip on the percept is loosened or broken.

HATHA YOGA

Even though the *Yoga-Sūtra* doesn't appear to be about hatha yoga, Patañjali's analysis of volition is essential to a safe and effective hatha practice. In his view, physical and mental actions are effects arising from conditioned, prior causes that are almost always imbued with suffering. It is difficult, therefore, to enact yogic movements of body and breath without unconsciously striving to feel good or eradicate some undesirable aspect of oneself or fortify the self or prolong life. Patañjali recognized that the causes of suffering arise from not seeing things as they are *(avidyā)*. Thus, seeing *(vidyā)* must be the primary orientation of a hatha yoga practice, lest its energies merely fuel the perpetually wanting self and its dissatisfactions.

In fact, hatha yoga practice may initially be driven to some extent by narcissism. After all, hatha yoga can appeal to us because of the powerful way it addresses some of the self's most cherished preoccupations—health, attractiveness, sexual energy, and longevity. When attachment to these properties lurks subliminally, seeding us with the urge to transcend phenomena like pain and fatigue simply in order to push the body beyond its barriers for its own sake, the potent hatha practice can be self-defeating and injurious. Even a practice that appears excruciatingly self-denying can be motivated by a subliminal need to adorn the self with the particular virtue of asceticism, itself but another form of adornment. Highly evolved teachers like Patañjali and the Buddha came to regard the ascetic impulse as a "near enemy" of awakening, seeming to be a support but actually hindering progress. With wise dedication and self-inquiry, though, hatha yoga can become a realization practice, illuminating the nature of our volitions and attachments, fostering radical self-acceptance, and weakening the grip of the self and its self-serving perspective.

Patañjali's yogic path may be described as traversing a series of perceptual thresholds. As powerful as hatha yoga practice can be, especially in establishing concentration and mindfulness, in general it lies beyond the threshold of stillness necessary for *samādhi*. That is not to say that effective hatha yoga practice can't produce a transparent, revelatory perspective regarding bodymind experience or bring about momentary epiphanies. Indeed, were it not for the fact that most of its movements require too much physical effort to be maintained for more than a few minutes, hatha yoga might well induce *samādhi* reliably. The processes of interiorization and calm are the same during *hatha-yogāsana-prāṇāyāma* as they are in Patañjali's *āsana-prāṇāyāma,* but the former are much more volitional in nature than the latter, which end in virtual nondoing. Thus the effects of *hatha-yogāsana-prāṇāyāma* occur at a different part of the continuum of psychosomatic activity, or *karma*. This is why hatha yoga most certainly can be meditation in action and a powerful vehicle in preparation for radical stillness but is not itself a *samādhi* practice.

Patañjali was a realist among idealists, his teaching a model of pragmatism. Absent of ceremoniousness or sentimentality, its program depends for its success solely on the energy and engagement the yogi brings to it. Awakening is not an intellectual event—nor, indeed, a mental activity of any kind—but instead emerges by itself when flesh and blood, mind and breath, are permeated more and more fully by the settling process, *nirodha*. For, though the mind plays a key role in holding on to the possibility of its own cessation and remembering the steps on the yogic path to cessation, discrimination *(viveka)* and wisdom *(prajñā)* cannot arise until cognitive and self-making activities cease; and even wisdom itself must settle if consciousness is to reflect ultimate, nonpersonal reality.

Thus Patañjali always returns to the prescription of nondoing as the most direct way for body and mind to unlearn what they think they know and thereby reset the course toward pure awareness. The trajectory of yoga takes us backward and inward through ourselves toward the clarity of primordial repose.

DUALISM AND NONDUALISM

The yogic path leads to realization, in which every aspect of being can be seen as it is. Each experience or attribute of the world—including oneself—is exposed as compound in nature, with all its particulars in flux. This is directly known by an awareness that is unconditioned and unchanging. From the yogic perspective, all suffering and confusion are seen through and neutralized by this realization. It is not necessary, therefore, to conceptualize, verbalize, or "make sense" of the experience in order to achieve freedom.

However, to communicate the possibility of liberation to others, to describe the processes of yoga, and to encourage others to try it, one must eventually do just that. While clearly recognizing the limits of the mind to know itself, Patañjali makes an appeal to the minds of his followers, and to all who would enter the yogic path, by offering them a conceptual model of reality. In that sense, the *Yoga-Sūtra* is a work of technical philosophy.

As soon as yoga enters the domain of philosophy, though, the mind must assert its special prerogative, however grandiose, to install itself as the locus of all knowledge. On that behalf, it must demand an answer to the following question: if awareness lies at the core of all experience, who is experiencing the awareness?

Awareness is much more vast than thought. While awareness easily accommodates all mental experience, the mind is too small a container for the contents of awareness. This seems to be because so many of its functions are dedicated to selecting and elaborating on the desirable and also filtering out or eliminating the undesirable. Even much of the mind's own content, such as the conditioned values that determine what is desirable or not, is internalized and hidden from conscious view to make room for efficient mental functioning. It is therefore impossible for the mind to swallow the whole stream of sensorimental phenomena, yet it is also difficult for it to grasp that it cannot. This would seem to be one of the factors that prevent the mind from accepting the knowable fact that awareness requires no experiencer or recipient.

In Patañjali's psychology, the mind is not the vehicle for the direct insight of realization, in which the world is seen as a dynamic flow of phenomena regarded by an unchanging, impersonal awareness. The qualities of these two domains, mind and awareness, seem so opposed that any analysis might well conclude that they are mutually exclusive, as his did, or reflect radically different aspects of the mind, as some Buddhist traditions maintain.

This conclusion reflects the mind's irresistible compulsion to reify and classify its experiences in relation to the self. It is in the nature of mind to sort things apart, compartmentalize them, and identify the laws governing their behavior and separateness. So the philosophical mind rightly sees dualism in Patañjali's isolation of awareness *(puruṣa)* from consciousness *(citta)* and nature *(prakṛti)*.

However, any philosophical analysis must also take into account Patañjali's negation of *puruṣa,* which he strips of any self properties whatsoever. Awareness itself has no attributes—no thought, action, cause, effect, temporality, materiality, or interaction with the world. One well might ask: Isn't seeing perhaps the fundamental, defining action of a self? Patañjali's reply is that the whole point of yoga is to recognize that seeing is not a self activity at all. In other words, the self stands before awareness, not behind it.

Another objection might also arise: Isn't *puruṣa*'s "coupling" to an individual being throughout life, dissolution, and rebirth a kind of interaction? Here it may be recalled that the apparent indivisibility *(saṃyoga)* with which awareness seems to be coupled to a being and its consciousness is a construct, not of awareness, but of consciousness. When the bustling consciousness apparatus *(citta)* is transformed through yogic stilling *(nirodha)* and thereby allowed to assume something like the luminous, propertyless nature of awareness, the appearance of coupling vanishes. This is not due to any action by *puruṣa,* which only *knows* action, but by the fact that *saṃyoga* is an artifact of *citta.* And it is this artifactual *saṃyoga*—the unconscious, deeply held notion that awareness and everything else must be of the same order—that makes *puruṣa*'s separateness *(kaivalya)* so jarring and difficult to accept. If this were not so, and the mind were able to see through the coupling of awareness and consciousness, liberation would be a far simpler matter.

Thus one must recognize that if the *yoga-darśana* is dualistic philosophy, it is a dualism that counterposes everything against virtually nothing. *Puruṣa* is not a substantial entity in any sense, being utterly devoid of qualities or essence. It neither adds to nor subtracts from what we know as the universe; it is just the knowing itself. Nonetheless, prior to the direct experience of discrimination, or *viveka,* one can't easily escape the mental conception that *puruṣa* and *prakṛti* are two different but comparable entities (see 2.26, commentary).

In practical terms, characterizing Patañjali's system as dualism hardly detracts from its primary purpose as a vehicle for realization and is not especially significant to the yogi. In fact, the most decisive transformation in the yogic process is the discovery of underlying phenomenal nonduality, which becomes visible with the arising of coalescence, or *samāpatti. Samāpatti* means "things falling together," and abiding in it steadily is *samādhi,* or "putting things together." When consciousness is becalmed to a mirrorlike reflectivity, all perceivable phenomena are seen for the first time to be unitary and nondual, though empty of seeing itself.

Once the conceptual mind has settled and integration *(samādhi)* has arisen, direct experience of the *puruṣa-prakṛti* distinction is similar to the nondual Buddhist insight of emptiness, or *śūnyatā*. Like Siddhartha Gautama, Patañjali found all world experience to be composed of a granular substrate of irreducible perceptual phenomena in constant flux—a *dharma* stream—in which he was unable to detect any subjectivity whatsoever. Nor could either teacher find any self or permanence in the sets of constituents conventionally experienced as the self. And since each and every datum of experience is the artifact of an impersonal consciousness, perception is never the reality of the object it represents. Unlike Gautama, though, Patañjali reified his insights by proposing a *puruṣa* explicitly exempted from the world of objects but all too easily mistaken for some kind of entity.

An intellectual picture of *puruṣa* may help one approach the true nature of awareness, in the way that a line on a road map may guide us toward our destination, even if it ultimately founders on our mental-linguistic inability to accommodate the seemingly paradoxical observations that awareness exists and that it cannot be located in any single sensation, thought, or feeling. A point of the *Yoga-Sūtra* is that concepts can be helpful as long as one keeps in mind that they belong to a different order of knowledge than seeing itself. Just as the dots on the map are nothing at all like a real city, all *puruṣa* concepts differ enormously from *puruṣa* realization. But while a city is so much more than a dot, *puruṣa* is vastly less. Every attempt by the self to confer its own apparent qualities on *puruṣa*—solidity, location, identity, subjectivity, essence, ownership—inflates *puruṣa* astronomically beyond what it is. This dilemma is the wedge that drives apart the words we use to describe knowing and embodiment.

For the reader of the *Yoga-Sūtra* who wants to use it for its primary purpose, as a guide to realization, therefore, it is critically important not to become identified with concepts of dualism or nondualism. Just as the line on the map is but a symbol of the actual highway, the *Yoga-Sūtra* is merely a conceptual analogue to the true yogic process, where all discursive activity must subside for wisdom to enter. To get anywhere at all, we must keep our eyes primarily not on the map but on the road itself.

That road leads us to a realm of profound insights—that all phenomena are in fact interconnected and impermanent, that the stuff of self is not other than the stuff of the world, and that the pure awareness regarding self and world is not colored by them. In the words of an ancient Indian saying, the lotus grows in muddy waters but shows no trace.

THE *YOGA-SŪTRA* IN LIGHT OF EARLY BUDDHISM

A comparative analysis of the *Yoga-Sūtra* and the Pali canon indicates that Siddhartha Gautama and Patañjali took similar approaches in their study of knowing and being and that they came to similar conclusions. Furthermore, the paths they proposed to end suffering were remarkably alike. Apart from the structures of their metaphysical systems, which are often at odds, their descriptions and prescriptions are generally compatible.

This should surprise no one familiar with the history of Indian religious thought. The teachings of the Buddha evolved directly from the brahmanical-Upaniṣadic traditions of yogic contemplation, purporting to clarify and improve on them, and are grounded in that cultural context. It is thus impossible not to view the Buddha's approach as yoga, and his realization can be seen as an invaluable clarification of those traditions. Likewise, operating in a cultural context at least six centuries distant from the Buddha's, Patañjali seems to have conscientiously practiced the dharma and achieved a profound realization. His account of it is comparable to the Buddha's but expressed in terms of the ascendant *sāṃkhya* worldview. The *Yoga-Sūtra* is also interspersed with occasional reproofs to then-popular Buddhist idealism, although it is not difficult to imagine Siddhartha Gautama himself reacting likewise. In any event, Patañjali's yoga evolved to a great extent from a Buddhistic approach that itself had been a development of brahmanical-Upaniṣadic yoga. This interweaving of influences is a characteristic feature of Indian philosophical thought.

While a detailed comparison of classical yoga and Buddhism lies beyond the scope of this book, it can be generally stated that from a technical standpoint, the foundational yogic practices of the two teachers are much the same, with certain differences of emphasis. Both methods focus on achieving cessation *(nirodha)* through the dispassionate observation of bodymind phenomena from an increasingly interiorized perspective, facilitated by sustained stillness. Each teacher gives special consideration to the energies of breathing, both as a compelling attentional anchor and as a vehicle for calming the bodymind. Furthermore, the establishment of bodymind repose and clarity represents the first stage of progressive dharmic investigation of knowing itself—an investigation much more thoroughly elaborated upon in the vast

Pali canon than in Patañjali's single surviving discourse. Likewise, Gautama skillfully extends the practice of mindfulness to the activities of daily life, an area not explicitly treated in the *Yoga-Sūtra.*

One of the central disagreements between the two traditions has to do with their somewhat different analyses of suffering. Each identifies four penetrating truths, although Patañjali doesn't link them together in a single *sūtra* grouping as the Buddha had. According to the first truth, suffering *(duḥkha)* is present in all experience, including selfhood. Second, *duḥkha* has a cause. Third, the suffering of *duḥkha* can be brought to an end. Finally, each teacher identifies a path to the end of suffering.

The first disparity between the teachings of the four truths is to be found in the identification of their cause. The Buddha located the source of *duḥkha* in what he called thirst (Skt: *tṛṣṇā;* Pali: *taṇhā*)—the primary urges informing all volition: to acquire, eliminate, or become. These "thirsts" are themselves conditioned on feelings *(vedanā)* as they arise and cannot therefore be thought of as absolute.

Similarly, Patañjali finds suffering in wanting *(rāga),* aversion *(dveṣa),* and becoming and sustaining a self *(asmitā; abhiniveśāḥ).* He also acknowledges that wanting and aversion are conditioned by sensory experience, but seems to attribute the survival urge to feeling like a self, which creates the self-reinforcing notion that the self is an entity of central and lasting importance, thereby requiring protection. These four causes of suffering *(kleśas),* however, are themselves predicated on a single primary cause: not seeing *(avidyā)* that awareness is distinct from the natural phenomena that appear to produce it. These include the senses, whose nonseeing products feel blended with the awareness seeing them. This projects an illusory sense of "I" that superimposes itself on the phenomenon of perceiving. The sense of "I" must be sustained because it is inaccurately experienced as the source of knowing and therefore mistakenly regarded as precious and irreplaceable. Yoga reveals the true source of knowing, the imperturbable *puruṣa,* rendering the self and its survival dramas irrelevant.

Just as the failure to recognize the difference between awareness and consciousness endows ultimately impersonal self-phenomena with an illusory sense of subjectivity, it likewise imparts a false feeling of thusness to objects. Each of the four secondary causes of suffering *(kleśas)* adds to an object by lending it properties that exist only in relation to the self illusion. Feeling like a self *(asmitā)* establishes the phantom self-presence, generating a feedback loop in which the self's "ownership" of experience magnifies its self-importance and makes it cling to its own existence *(abhiniveśā)*. Wanting *(rāga)* infuses the object with the property of necessity in regard to the self, while aversion *(dveṣa)* imbues it with repulsiveness and intolerability. In this way all objects, including self experience, are amplified and prolonged far beyond their intrinsic mutability.

Although Gautama named "thirst" as the primary cause of suffering in the second Noble Truth, he also taught, especially in the *Mahā-satipaṭṭhāna-sutta* (Pali, "great discourse on the establishing of mindfulness"), that the purpose of clarifying the nature of phenomena was to recognize and extinguish the "fires" of wanting *(rāga)*, aversion *(dveṣa)*, and confusion *(moha)* that inflame all experience.

Patañjali was not an idealist along the lines of certain of his Buddhist contemporaries. Objects have a real existence, he argued, and don't vanish when we turn from them (4.16). It's just that the apparently foundational properties of an object—projected onto ordinary perception in ever changing proportions of light, motion, and mass *(guṇas)*—are actually nonessential. And all of these seemingly foundational properties arise purely in relation to a self that is itself an empty construct. While this view clashes with the more radically inclusive Mahāyāna conception of emptiness and subjectivity that was developing in Patañjali's day, it is quite similar to Siddhartha Gautama's teaching.

That the appearances of phenomena are so chronically misperceived is indicative of the coarseness afflicting our everyday perceptual modes, which can be transcended through yogic training. Like the Buddha, Patañjali emphasizes that wanting, aversion, and self-making are conditioned and relative and that the very contents that give rise to them are, when viewed in the proper light, also the ground of liberation from them (2.18). From his perspective, once experience can be seen accurately *(vidyā),* its surfaces become the very mirror that reflects the freedom *(kaivalya)* of awareness to itself. And the third truth enumerated by each teacher is that this illuminated perspective arises with the cessation *(nirodha-samāpatti)* of all volitional physical and mental activity erupting from these urges. Patañjali's teaching, rendered in a *sāṃkhya* cast, offers considerable detail regarding the process of imprinting, storing, and releasing the latent impressions *(saṃskāras)* of internal and external experience, and he implicates this process as the mechanism through which suffering perpetuates itself.

Regarding their respective eightfold paths to the end of suffering, Patañjali takes a somewhat different approach from his predecessor, laying out the path as a series of thresholds at which yoking occurs. While progress on the yogic path constitutes or depends on elements also found in the Buddha's Noble Eightfold Path, Patañjali doesn't specifically assign them "limb" *(aṅgam)* status. These include the will to practice *(abhyāsa)* and to let go *(vairāgya),* corresponding roughly to the Buddha's right effort to sustain wholesome states of mind and eliminate the unwholesome (see also 2.33, 2.34). While the Buddha devotes extensive attention to the particular qualities of right speech, livelihood, thought, and understanding, Patañjali uses his eight-part formulation to focus on elements more explicitly related to the successively interiorized frontiers of yoking, such as internal disciplines *(niyamas),* posture *(āsana),* breath *(prāṇāyāma),* withdrawal of the senses *(pratyāhāra),* and the "perfect discipline" of *saṃyama.* Having done so, he then elaborates on some of the qualities mentioned by the Buddha, including the effects of wholesome thought and the nature of wisdom *(prajñā).* But as mentioned above, it is the Buddha who offers the more detailed path of investigation.

As similar as the Buddhist and yogic paths are, one aspect of their metaphysical models is difficult to reconcile. Siddhartha Gautama, living at a time of Upaniṣadic influence, carefully but repeatedly rejected the Vedantic notion that there is any changeless soul entity (*ātman*) abiding in the midst of the phenomenal world and its flux. This would seem to put him at odds with Patañjali, at least as interpreted in the traditional Vedantic style most prevalent today. Interestingly, though, Patañjali's *puruṣa* itself differs from the Vedantic *ātman* to some extent. The latter is definitively affiliated with an individual *(jiva)* but is seen through realization not to be different from the universal matrix *(brahman),* which is both absolute and relative, manifesting as the world through the play of the lord *īśvara.* For Patañjali, though, *īśvara* is a *puruṣa,* and *puruṣas* do not interact with the world, much less set it in motion with their play. It is not even clear if a *puruṣa* is individual, submerged though it is in the identity of an individuated consciousness. For Patañjali, *puruṣa* is simply the impersonal awareness principle and nothing more. This may still be at odds with the Buddha's teaching that all phenomena are without self (Pali: *sabbe dhammā anattā*), which presumably includes the conditioned realm of experience and also the unconditioned *nirvāṇa* (Pali: *nibbāṇa*) One might well ask, though, What is it that knows the nature of unsatisfactoriness, impermanence, selflessness, and *nirvāṇa*? Both Patañjali and Siddhartha Gautama would agree that nothing resembling a self, or even an "it," is involved.

THE *YOGA-SŪTRA* IN LIGHT OF CONTEMPORARY SCIENTIFIC KNOWLEDGE

Perhaps the greatest difference between modern and ancient practice has to do with the underlying goals of meditation then and now. In earlier times yogis traveled the path of awakening with two intertwined objectives. The first was to achieve freedom from suffering by seeing beyond the appearances of consciousness and realizing pure awareness. The second goal of practice was to unlock the secrets of the phenomenal world: by cultivating the powers of concentration and observation, yogis came to a profounder sense of what the world actually was and how its objects behaved. This second domain of yogic exploration, indivisible from the first, was scientific, investigative, and descriptive, encompassing what is now called psychology as well as aspects of physical science and philosophy. It is also phenomenological—based primarily on what can be directly experienced by awareness of sensory and mental experience per se, rather than known through inference. While Patañjali's *Yoga-Sūtra* is mainly about freedom from suffering, it also attempts to describe what and how the world is, largely in accordance with the *sāṃkhya* view.

Patañjali makes a point of asserting, in 4.16, that the world is objectively real, even though appearing differently to each individual observer. In light of that assertion, though, we must acknowledge that much more is known about certain aspects of the world now than in Patañjali's time and that this knowledge was attained largely through scientific inference. Patañjali certainly regarded such knowledge as valid and potentially useful in the pursuit of realization.

Regardless of one's respect for the depth of Patañjali's phenomenological inquiry, it might be difficult, and perhaps unwise, for the modern yogi to embrace the entirety of the *Yoga-Sūtra*'s scientific paradigm uncritically. For example, we now know that most natural phenomena occur beyond the range of human perception. The greater part of nature unfolds in the form of events that are either too slow, too fast, too great, or too tiny to observe directly. For example, our senses alone cannot detect the growth of most things, whether mountains or trees or our own fingernails. Meanwhile, particles, meteors, and waves of ultraviolet light fly by us, no more perceptible than hummingbird wings. We fail even to sense that we are standing atop a planet or that we are composed of molecules, let alone atoms.

Human beings today are constantly reminded that much if not most of existence lies beyond our senses. Our culture is deeply informed by knowledge of things that were unknown in ancient times. Most children, even small ones, have seen pictures of galaxies and DNA, for example—images containing information that surely would have interested Patañjali and influenced his views. Because we know something of the inconceivable power of radio telescopes and electron microscopes, our internalized sense of our own organic perceptual range is drastically diminished compared with that of the ancients.

Patañjali asserts that no two people see an object in exactly the same way and recognizes that much of nature is unmanifest and not directly knowable. Nonetheless, he concludes that matter is undergoing precisely the same sort of transformations that he observes in regard to consciousness *(citta-vṛtti)*. The illusion of seeing the world and its constituent parts as operating under the same processes as the consciousness that represents them may have been inescapable for ancient observers who lacked an internalized skepticism about the range of their yogically clarified perceptions. Phenomenology was therefore conflated with naturalism. While this notion feels right and may satisfy any idealistic longing one might have for the possibility of omniscience, it no longer conforms to scientific understanding.

Even if contemporary physical models have eclipsed the *sāṃkhya-yoga* view in certain respects, the yogis were correct in concluding that consciousness was made of the same stuff as everything else. This alone was a remarkable achievement. Furthermore, Patañjali's findings about the impersonality of conscious processes are difficult to refute, based as they are not on inference but on direct knowledge, seeing through the appearances of the self and the world and watching their distinctions dissolve.

If current scientific understanding makes it difficult to accept the *sāṃkhya* view, shared by Patañjali, that awareness is other than nature, our burgeoning knowledge of the brain's architecture and function goes a long way toward explaining why, in an important sense, Patañjali's description might feel correct. While all forms of awareness are now attributed to neuronal activity in the brain and the rest of the central and peripheral nervous systems, awareness per se does not seem to reside in the neurons themselves but in the concerted patterns of energy they evoke. Even a simple representation involves inconceivably complex sequences of neuronal excitation, thrown up in an array something like a hologram—but not actually thrown up in an identifiable location. Although the succession of representation moments Patañjali deconstructs might roughly be compared to the frames of a movie, there is no theater anywhere in the brain, in fact, nor even a screen on which these patterns actually flicker.

Thus, in a sense, all knowing is truly empty of essence or locus, as in both Buddhist and yogic perspectives. Every aspect of experience is encoded and reiterated, not in the neurons themselves, but in their collective patterns of firing. This gives the modern yogi a more solid foundation for understanding Patañjali's view of awareness and also the concept of latent impressions, or *saṃskāras*. And as the nervous system becomes more refined and sensitive to its own inner workings, it can begin to intuit how experience is stored in itself—and then reemerges in the form of new thoughts and actions conditioned by the old—by sensing the sequential nature of phenomena rather than locating a precise material topography.

Thus it may not be necessary to endorse the notion of rebirth, grounded in the prevailing beliefs of Patañjali's culture, in order to accept his view of cause and effect. One can clearly detect the operation of the *karma-saṃskāra-karma* cycle without having to enter into metaphysical speculations regarding a latent impression's storage as energy or its survival beyond death. Furthermore, the appearance of strikingly individual traits in even the very young might be more attributable to hereditary or congenital factors than to the transmigration of seeds sown in a previous life. The science of genetics helps to account for many aspects of life that had previously been attributed to rebirth, although the influence of our thoughts and actions—our *karma*—on the hereditary legacy we pass on to our children is still not well understood today.

Many celebrated and influential yogis from ancient times to the present—most famously, the Buddha—have concluded that one can awaken fully without having to engage in metaphysical speculation at all. Likewise one might travel the yogic path end to end, arriving at its conclusive liberation without having had to consider—much less exercise—most if not all the shamanic powers enumerated in chapter 3. Patañjali himself places the attainment of discrimination between *puruṣa* and *prakṛti* above other powers, which might be viewed as distractions from the true goal of yoga, liberation. And discrimination cannot be inferred—it must be experienced directly, even by cognitive scientists.

But the question remains: Is *puruṣa* veridical or merely a neural representation? The very word *representation* implies that something is being displayed to something else, yet pure awareness feels irreducible. In discrimination there is a sense of *puruṣa's* ultimacy, of its being the coreless core of reality, the eye behind the eye. Patañjali describes *puruṣa-īśvara* as unconditioned by cause and effect and universal rather than self-generated, so there can be no doubt that he regarded awareness as utterly nonphysical. Yet it may simply be that it is just the matrix of consciousness, invisible unless all cortical representation ceases, settled to the point where it ceases to be colored by any constructive or associative activity at all. Then, and only then, would it seem as if awareness were free *(kaivalya)* of the innumerable attributes and mandates of the world as ordinarily reflected in the cortex's encyclopedically conditioned perspective.

In any case, directly knowing the way things are remains a very different matter than making sense of them. As in music, where silently analyzing the score of a symphony might be instructive but could never replace the actual sounds ringing in the ears, yogic practice must supersede theory.

Kriyā-yoga, the Path of Action

Just as the acquisition of supernormal powers can hardly be regarded as the ultimate goal of the *Yoga-Sūtra,* neither are its purpose and value primarily intellectual or scientific. It is unlikely that Patañjali intended his students to dwell on its philosophical assertions, except insofar as they provided support for the yoking process. Thus the *Yoga-Sūtra* emphasizes *kriyā-yoga,* or yogic action, whose three components are intensity *(tapas),* self-study *(svādhyāya),* and orientation *(praṇidhāna)* toward *īśvara,* the divine exemplar of pure awareness.

Ideally, in light of the fact that it was probably composed as a kind of textbook, the work is best understood and utilized in the context of an interactive teacher-student relationship. Unfortunately, yoga teachers whose knowledge and personal realization would qualify them for this purpose are rare. This is not necessarily different from the way things were for the yogis of antiquity. Deeply realized sages who are also able to teach effectively have probably been in short supply throughout history and may well remain so. Besides, the qualities that Patañjali prized—discipline, self-study, and surrender—are highly individual and must arise from personal initiative. And despite the need for guidance, one ultimately treads the path alone.

Of these three valuable qualities, self-study, or *svādhyāya,* is the actual way that we can understand and assimilate Patañjali's program today in our own lives. Like the rest of the yogic system, *svādhyāya* is a unitary process with several different, interdependent aspects. The first involves regular study of the *sūtras,* with an attitude of openness and humility. While never forgetting that the *Yoga-Sūtra* and other wisdom teachings are human works and therefore inevitably imperfect, one must acknowledge that their limitations may not be truly verifiable until their truths are clearly grasped. This is particularly true of teachings that emphasize action over theory. Much practice and reflection are required over time if the subtle meanings of many yogic concepts are to come clear.

The second element of *svādhyāya* is a compassionate but ruthless daily survey of one's own thoughts and deeds. In what may be a nod to the diverse pantheon in his day, Patañjali mentions that study, and perhaps chanting, of the *sūtras* "deepens communion with one's personal deity" (2.44). More telling, however, is his repeated emphasis throughout the *Yoga-Sūtra* on the importance of studying oneself. Without rigorous self-examination it is all too easy to fall into patterns of internal and external behavior that impede our emergent awakening and perpetuate old cycles of misunderstanding and suffering. As Patañjali points out in regard to the *yamas* and *niyamas,* when one's life comes to conform to them, no one benefits more than oneself, even though they can exert powerful effects on other beings as well.

The third aspect of *svādhyāya* consists in carefully comparing the *Yoga-Sūtra's* descriptions of consciousness with our own experience. This and other ancient yogic and Buddhist texts detail levels of insight that are chiefly stabilized through yogic practice and have never since been described as thoroughly or well. Modern languages have few or no equivalents that can accommodate the pregnant fullness of many Sanskrit and Pali terms. For example, to understand a word like *samāpatti,* one must tread the same path as the ancient yogis, carefully observing one's body and breath movements until the phenomenon of coalescence becomes palpable. It is this aspect of self-study that fleshes out Patañjali's concepts and also reveals the inadequacy of all language, even the highly evolved tongues of Sanskrit and Pali, to convey the essential truths of yoga.

In the final aspect of *svādhyāya,* one undertakes to follow the directives of the *Yoga-Sūtra* faithfully, even as they lead one away from everything one might have thought of as being fully alive. The entire trajectory of the yogic process arcs away from what we thought life was all about, and toward a degree of stillness and absorption that the mind can't help but associate with vacuity. Not only do we forswear indulgence in food, drink, sex, and material enjoyment, we even stop moving and breathing altogether for long periods, ceasing to react with anything but openness even to the most compelling sensations or emotions. No longer do we permit ourselves to wallow in dazzling arrays of thought churned out by our spectacularly prolific minds, nor do we identify with any of their contents at all, even though we had previously experienced it all as "ours."

Naturally, the self cannot suffer this yoking gladly. From its worldly perspective, these developments must result in a barren mentality, stripped of the juicy vividness that only thought and desire would seem to provide. However, yogic action takes one beyond the solipsism of the self. As the bodymind settles, one begins to see with stunning clarity that all experience is seeded with the causes of suffering. These seeds lie below the surface of awareness but germinate continuously in one's thoughts and actions, thereby reseeding the ground of one's being with wanting, aversion, egoism, and a clinging to life. Having seen this, one is ready for freedom from the self's narcissistic autocracy.

Needless to say, the self is resistant to any approach that might involve a true letting go of attachments. Even with the prospect of imminent awakening, Patañjali tells us in 3.52 and 4.27, the self is poised to assert its privileges of ownership on all experience. After all, if realization is going to happen, "I" and "mine" don't want to miss it.

Thus, to effect change requires energy, converted to the heat of intense discipline, or *tapas*. In Patañjali's formulation of yogic action, or *kriyā-yoga,* one enforces yoking through *tapas,* generated at many levels of human experience. In daily life, this means placing realization at the center of one's priorities, not only by practicing constantly and with complete engagement to enter the stilling process *(nirodha)* through daily meditation, but also by bringing every aspect of one's work and relationships into alignment with the awakening process. In the stilling practice, *tapas* is the energy fueling both the persistent returning to focus *(abhyāsa)* and the willingness to see all experience with clarity instead of reaction *(vairāgya)*. At physiological and energetic levels, *tapas* is both the heat that rises from the fires of bodily purification, especially as elaborated in later tantric technologies like hatha yoga, and the "heat of surrender" when we open our valves wide to the stream of momentary experience. Each time we can observe without reacting as an impulse to think or act out according to conditioned and well-worn patterns of suffering arises, we are in effect practicing a small but significant austerity that unlocks immeasurable energy. And only by dying to what we thought we were can we enter the sublime realm of what truly is.

The supreme goal of *kriyā-yoga,* at last, is to recognize that a transcendent, timeless awareness underlies all phenomenal experience. If anything in existence can be called divine, it is the natural perfection of this witness that sees through the illusory projections of consciousness. Conceived by Patañjali as both divine and universal—*īśvara* and *puruṣa*—pure seeing is the sacred shore that all inward journeys hope to reach. As we embark on our journey, we can take sustenance and direction from Patañjali's words—for those who seek liberation wholeheartedly, realization is near. Collecting the strands of ancient yogic knowledge, he has woven a thread—a *sūtra*—that traces the path to freedom. In taking up his thread and following it, we find that it leads not away but straight back to the heart of the self.

APPENDIX A

THE YOGA-SŪTRA IN ENGLISH

Chapter 1. Integration

1 Now, the teachings of yoga.

2 Yoga is to still the patterning of consciousness.

3 Then pure awareness can abide in its very nature.

4 Otherwise awareness takes itself to be the patterns of consciousness.

5 There are five types of patterns, including both hurtful and benign.

6 They are right perception, misperception, conceptualization, deep sleep, and remembering.

7 Right perception arises from direct observation, inference, or the words of others.

8 Misperception is false knowledge, not based on what actually is.

9 Conceptualization is based on linguistic knowledge, not contact with real things.

10 Deep sleep is a pattern grounded in the perception that nothing exists.

11 Remembering is the retention of experiences.

12 Both practice and nonreaction are required to still the patterning of consciousness.

13 Practice is the sustained effort to rest in that stillness.

14 This practice becomes firmly rooted when it is cultivated skillfully and continuously for a long time.

15 As for nonreaction, one can recognize that it has been fully achieved when no attachment arises in regard to anything at all, whether perceived directly or learned.

16 When the ultimate level of nonreaction has been reached, pure awareness can clearly see itself as independent from the fundamental qualities of nature.

17 At first the stilling process is accompanied by four kinds of cognition: analytical thinking, insight, bliss, and feeling like a self.

18 Later, after one practices steadily to bring all thought to a standstill, these four kinds of cognition fall away, leaving only a store of latent impressions in the depth memory.

19 These latent impressions incline one to be reborn after one leaves the body at death and is dissolved in nature.

20 For all others, faith, energy, mindfulness, integration, and wisdom form the path to realization.

21 For those who seek liberation wholeheartedly, realization is near.

22 How near depends on whether the practice is mild, moderate, or intense.

23 Realization may also come if one is oriented toward the ideal of pure awareness, *īśvara*.

24 *Īśvara* is a distinct, incorruptible form of pure awareness, utterly independent of cause and effect and lacking any store of latent impressions.

25 Its independence makes this awareness an incomparable source of omniscience.

26 Existing beyond time, *īśvara* was also the ideal of the ancients.

27 *Īśvara* is represented by a sound, *ōm*.

28 Through repetition its meaning becomes clear.

29 Then interiorization develops and obstacles fall away.

30 Sickness, apathy, doubt, carelessness, laziness, sexual indulgence, delusion, lack of progress, and inconstancy are all distractions that, by stirring up consciousness, act as barriers to stillness.

31 When they do, one may experience distress, depression, or the inability to maintain steadiness of posture or breathing.

32 One can subdue these distractions by working with any one of the following principles of practice.

33 Consciousness settles as one radiates friendliness, compassion, delight, and equanimity toward all things, whether pleasant or painful, good or bad.

34 Or by pausing after breath flows in or out.

35 Or by steadily observing as new sensations materialize.

36 Or when experiencing thoughts that are luminous and free of sorrow.

37 Or by focusing on things that do not inspire attachment.

38 Or by reflecting on insights culled from sleep and dreaming.

39 Or through meditative absorption in any desired object.

40 One can become fully absorbed in any object, whether vast or infinitesimal.

41 As the patterning of consciousness subsides, a transparent way of seeing, called coalescence, saturates consciousness; like a jewel, it reflects equally whatever lies before it—whether subject, object, or act of perceiving.

42 So long as conceptual or linguistic knowledge pervades this transparency, it is called coalescence with thought.

43 At the next stage, called coalescence beyond thought, objects cease to be colored by memory; now formless, only their essential nature shines forth.

44 In the same way, coalesced contemplation of subtle objects is described as reflective or reflection-free.

45 Subtle objects can be traced back to their origin in undifferentiated nature.

46 These four kinds of coalesced contemplation—with thought, beyond thought, reflective, reflection-free—are called integration that bears seeds of latent impressions.

47 In the lucidity of coalesced, reflection-free contemplation, the nature of the self becomes clear.

48 The wisdom that arises in that lucidity is unerring.

49 Unlike insights acquired through inference or teachings, this wisdom has as its object the actual distinction between pure awareness and consciousness.

50 It generates latent impressions that prevent the activation of other impressions.

51 When even these cease to arise and the patterning of consciousness is completely stilled, integration bears no further seeds.

Chapter 2. The Path to Realization

1 Yogic action has three components—discipline, self-study, and orientation toward the ideal of pure awareness.

2 Its purposes are to disarm the causes of suffering and achieve integration.

3 The causes of suffering are not seeing things as they are, the sense of "I," attachment, aversion, and clinging to life.

4 Not seeing things as they are is the field where the other causes of suffering germinate, whether dormant, activated, intercepted, or weakened.

5 Lacking this wisdom, one mistakes that which is impermanent, impure, distressing, or empty of self for permanence, purity, happiness, and self.

6 The sense of "I" ascribes selfhood to pure awareness by identifying it with the senses.

7 Attachment is a residue of pleasant experience.

8 Aversion is a residue of suffering.

9 Clinging to life is instinctive and self-perpetuating, even for the wise.

10 In their subtle form, these causes of suffering are subdued by seeing where they come from.

11 In their gross form, as patterns of consciousness, they are subdued through meditative absorption.

12 The causes of suffering are the root source of actions; each action deposits latent impressions deep in the mind, to be activated and experienced later in this birth or lie hidden awaiting a future one.

13 So long as this root source exists, its contents will ripen into a birth, a life, and experience.

14 This life will be marked by delight or anguish, in proportion to those good or bad actions that created its store of latent impressions.

15 The wise see suffering in all experience, whether from the anguish of impermanence or from latent impressions

laden with suffering or from incessant conflict as the fundamental qualities of nature vie for ascendancy.

16 But suffering that has not yet arisen can be prevented.

17 The preventable cause of all this suffering is the apparent indivisibility of pure awareness and what it regards.

18 What awareness regards, namely the phenomenal world, embodies the qualities of luminosity, activity, and inertia; it includes oneself, composed of both elements and the senses; and it is the ground for both sensual experience and liberation.

19 All orders of being—undifferentiated, differentiated, indistinct, distinct—are manifestations of the fundamental qualities of nature.

20 Pure awareness is just seeing itself; although pure, it usually appears to operate through the perceiving mind.

21 In essence, the phenomenal world exists to reveal this truth.

22 Once that happens, the phenomenal world no longer appears as such, though it continues to exist as a common reality for everyone else.

23 It is by virtue of the apparent indivisibility of awareness and the phenomenal world that the latter seems to possess the former's powers.

24 Not seeing things as they are is the cause of this phenomenon.

25 With realization, the appearance of indivisibility vanishes, revealing that awareness is free and untouched by phenomena.

26 The apparent indivisibility of seeing and the seen can be eradicated by cultivating uninterrupted discrimination between awareness and what it regards.

27 At the ultimate level of discrimination, wisdom extends to all seven aspects of nature.

28 When the components of yoga are practiced, impurities dwindle; then the light of understanding can shine forth, illuminating the way to discriminative awareness.

29 The eight components of yoga are external discipline, internal discipline, posture, breath regulation, concentration, meditative absorption, and integration.

30 The five external disciplines are not harming, truthfulness, not stealing, celibacy, and not being acquisitive.

31 These universals, transcending birth, place, era, or circumstance, constitute the great vow of yoga.

32 The five internal disciplines are bodily purification, contentment, intense discipline, self-study, and dedication to the ideal of yoga.

33 Unwholesome thoughts can be neutralized by cultivating wholesome ones.

34 We ourselves may act upon unwholesome thoughts, such as wanting to harm someone, or we may cause or condone them in others; unwholesome thoughts may arise from greed, anger, or delusion; they may be mild, moderate, or extreme; but they never cease to ripen into ignorance and suffering. This is why one must cultivate wholesome thoughts.

35 Being firmly grounded in nonviolence creates an atmosphere in which others can let go of their hostility.

36 For those grounded in truthfulness, every action and its consequences are imbued with truth.

37 For those who have no inclination to steal, the truly precious is at hand.

38 The chaste acquire vitality.

39 Freedom from wanting unlocks the real purpose of existence.

40 With bodily purification, one's body ceases to be compelling, likewise contact with others.

41 Purification also brings about clarity, happiness, concentration, mastery of the senses, and capacity for self-awareness.

42 Contentment brings unsurpassed joy.

43 As intense discipline burns up impurities, the body and its senses become supremely refined.

44 Self-study deepens communion with one's personal deity.

45 Through orientation toward the ideal of pure awareness, one can achieve integration.

46 The postures of meditation should embody steadiness and ease.

47 This occurs as all effort relaxes and coalescence arises, revealing that the body and the infinite universe are indivisible.

48 Then one is no longer disturbed by the play of opposites.

49 With effort relaxing, the flow of inhalation and exhalation can be brought to a standstill; this is called breath regulation.

50 As the movement patterns of each breath—inhalation, exhalation, lull—are observed as to duration, number, and area of focus, breath becomes spacious and subtle.

51 As realization dawns, the distinction between breathing in and out falls away.

52 Then the veil lifts from the mind's luminosity.

53 And the mind is now fit for concentration.

54 When consciousness interiorizes by uncoupling from external objects, the senses do likewise; this is called withdrawal of the senses.

55 Then the senses reside utterly in the service of realization.

Chapter 3. The Extraordinary Powers

1 Concentration locks consciousness on a single area.

2 In meditative absorption, the entire perceptual flow is aligned with that object.

3 When only the essential nature of the object shines forth, as if formless, integration has arisen.

4 Concentration, absorption, and integration regarding a single object compose the perfect discipline of consciousness.

5 Once the perfect discipline of consciousness is mastered, wisdom dawns.

6 Perfect discipline is mastered in stages.

7 These three components—concentration, absorption, and integration—are more interiorized than the preceding five.

8 Even these three are external to integration that bears no seeds.

9 The transformation toward total stillness occurs as new latent impressions fostering cessation arise to prevent the activation of distractive, stored ones and moments of stillness begin to permeate consciousness.

10 These latent impressions help consciousness flow from one tranquil moment to the next.

11 Consciousness is transformed toward integration as distractions dwindle and focus arises.

12 In other words, consciousness is transformed toward focus as continuity develops between arising and subsiding perceptions.

13 Consciousness evolves along the same three lines—form, time span, and condition—as the elements and the senses.

14 The substrate is unchanged, whether before, during, or after it takes a given form.

15 These transformations appear to unfold the way they do because consciousness is a succession of distinct patterns.

16 Observing these three axes of change—form, time span, and condition—with perfect discipline yields insight into the past and future.

17 Word, meaning, and perception tend to get lumped together, each confused with the others; focusing on the distinctions between them with perfect discipline yields insight into the language of all beings.

18 Directly observing latent impressions with perfect discipline yields insight into previous births.

19 Focusing with perfect discipline on the perceptions of another yields insight into that person's consciousness.

20 But not insight regarding the object of those perceptions, since the object itself is not actually present in that person's consciousness.

21 When the body's form is observed with perfect discipline, it becomes invisible: the eye is disengaged from incoming light, and the power to perceive is suspended.

22 Likewise, through perfect discipline other percepts—sound, smell, taste, touch—can be made to disappear.

23 The effects of action may be immediate or slow in coming; observing one's actions with perfect discipline, or studying omens, yields insight into death.

24 Focusing with perfect discipline on friendliness, compassion, delight, and equanimity, one is imbued with their energies.

25 Focusing with perfect discipline on the powers of an elephant or other entities, one acquires those powers.

26 Being absorbed in the play of the mind's luminosity yields insight about the subtle, hidden, and distant.

27 Focusing with perfect discipline on the sun yields insight about the universe.

28 Focusing with perfect discipline on the moon yields insight about the stars' positions.

29 Focusing with perfect discipline on the polestar yields insight about the stars' movements.

30 Focusing with perfect discipline on the navel energy center yields insight about the organization of the body.

31 Focusing with perfect discipline on the pit of the throat eradicates hunger and thirst.

32 Focusing with perfect discipline on the "tortoise channel," one cultivates steadiness.

33 Focusing with perfect discipline on the light in the crown of the head, one acquires the perspective of the perfected ones.

34 Or, all these accomplishments may be realized in a flash of spontaneous illumination.

35 Focusing with perfect discipline on the heart, one understands the nature of consciousness.

36 Experience consists of perceptions in which the luminous aspect of the phenomenal world is mistaken for absolutely pure awareness. Focusing with perfect discipline on the different properties of each yields insight into the nature of pure awareness.

37 Following this insight, the senses—hearing, feeling, seeing, tasting, smelling—may suddenly be enhanced.

38 These sensory gifts may feel like attainments, but they distract one from integration.

39 By relaxing one's attachment to the body, and becoming profoundly sensitive to its currents, consciousness can enter another's body.

40 By mastering the flow of energy in the head and neck, one can walk through water, mud, thorns, and other obstacles without touching down but rather floating over them.

41 By mastering the flow of energy through the solar plexus, one becomes radiant.

42 By focusing with perfect discipline on the way sound travels through the ether, one acquires divine hearing.

43 By focusing with perfect discipline on the body's relationship to the ether and developing coalesced contemplation on the lightness of cotton, one can travel through space.

44 When consciousness completely disengages from externals—the "great disembodiment"—then the veil lifts from the mind's luminosity.

45 By observing the aspects of matter—gross, subtle, intrinsic, relational, purposive—with perfect discipline, one masters the elements.

46 Then extraordinary faculties appear, including the power to shrink to the size of an atom, as the body attains perfection, transcending physical law.

47 This perfection includes beauty, grace, strength, and the firmness of a diamond.

48 By observing the various aspects of the sense organs—their processes of perception, intrinsic natures, identification as self, interconnectedness, purposes—with perfect discipline, one masters them.

49 Then, free from the constraints of their organs, the senses perceive with the quickness of the mind, no longer in the sway of the phenomenal world.

50 Once one just sees the distinction between pure awareness and the luminous aspect of the phenomenal world, all conditions are known and mastered.

51 When one is unattached even to this omniscience and mastery, the seeds of suffering wither and awareness knows it stands alone.

52 Even if the exalted beckon, one must avoid attachment and pride, or suffering will recur.

53 Focusing with perfect discipline on the succession of moments in time yields insight born of discrimination.

54 This insight allows one to tell things apart that, through similarities of origin, feature, or position, had seemed continuous.

55 In this way discriminative insight deconstructs all of the phenomenal world's objects and conditions, setting them apart from pure awareness.

56 Once the luminosity and transparency of consciousness have become as distilled as pure awareness, they can reflect the freedom of awareness back to itself.

Chapter 4. Freedom

1 The attainments brought about by integration may also arise at birth, through the use of herbs, from intonations, or through austerity.

2 Being delivered into a new form comes about when natural forces overflow.

3 The transformation into this form or that is not driven by the causes proximate to it, just oriented by them, the way a farmer diverts a stream for irrigation.

4 Feeling like a self is the frame that orients consciousness toward individuation.

5 A succession of consciousnesses, generating a vast array of distinctive perceptions, appears to consolidate into one individual consciousness.

6 Once consciousness is fixed in meditative absorption, it no longer contributes to the store of latent impressions.

7 The actions of a realized yogi transcend good and evil, whereas the actions of others may be good or evil or both.

8 Each action comes to fruition by coloring latent impressions according to its quality—good, evil, or both.

9 Because the depth memory and its latent impressions are of a piece, their dynamic of cause and effect flows uninterruptedly across the demarcations of birth, place, and time.

10 They have always existed, because the will to exist is eternal.

11 Since its cause, effect, basis, and object are inseparable, a latent impression disappears when they do.

12 The past and future are immanent in an object, existing as different sectors in the same flow of experiential forms.

13 The characteristics of these sectors, whether manifest or subtle, are imparted by the fundamental qualities of nature.

14 Their transformations tend to blur together, imbuing each new object with a quality of substantiality.

15 People perceive the same object differently, as each person's perception follows a separate path from another's.

16 But the object is not dependent on either of those perceptions; if it were, what would happen to it when nobody was looking?

17 An object is known only by a consciousness it has colored; otherwise it is not known.

18 Patterns of consciousness are always known by pure awareness, their ultimate, unchanging witness.

19 Consciousness is seen not by its own light but by awareness.

20 Furthermore, consciousness and its object cannot be perceived at once.

21 If consciousness were perceived by itself instead of by awareness, the chain of such perceptions would regress infinitely, imploding memory.

22 Once it is stilled, though, consciousness comes to resemble unchanging awareness and can reflect itself being perceived.

23 Then consciousness can be colored by both awareness and the phenomenal world, thereby fulfilling all its purposes.

24 Even when colored by countless latent traits, consciousness, like all compound phenomena, has another purpose—to serve awareness.

25 As soon as one can distinguish between consciousness and awareness, the ongoing construction of the self ceases.

26 Consciousness, now oriented to this distinction, can gravitate toward freedom—the fully integrated knowledge that awareness is independent of nature.

27 Any gaps in discriminating awareness allow distracting thoughts to emerge from the store of latent impressions.

28 These distractions can be subdued, as the causes of suffering were, by tracing them back to their origin, or through meditative absorption.

29 One who regards even the most exalted states disinterestedly, discriminating continuously between pure awareness and the phenomenal world, enters the final stage of integration, in which nature is seen to be a cloud of irreducible experiential forms.

30 This realization extinguishes both the causes of suffering and the cycle of cause and effect.

31 Once all the layers and imperfections concealing truth have been washed away, insight is boundless, with little left to know.

32 Then the seamless flow of reality, its transformations colored by the fundamental qualities, begins to break down, fulfilling the true mission of consciousness.

33 One can see that the flow is actually a series of discrete events, each corresponding to the merest instant of time, in which one form becomes another.

34 Freedom is at hand when the fundamental qualities of nature, each of their transformations witnessed at the moment of its inception, are recognized as irrelevant to pure awareness; it stands alone, grounded in its very nature, the power of pure seeing. That is all.

APPENDIX B

About the Text and Translation

For two millennia the *Yoga-Sūtra* has been an essential resource for anyone traveling the yogic path to enlightenment, and Patañjali's analysis of consciousness and awareness has been available to the West since the nineteenth century. Nonetheless, the *Yoga-Sūtra* is neither widely nor well understood, for several reasons.

In the first place, its historical and philosophical origins are unclear. According to the current scholarly consensus, it was composed somewhere in India around the second or third century CE. It may well be the work of an unknown man or woman who was given the already illustrious Patañjali name posthumously. There are indications that some of the *Yoga-Sūtra* is a transmission of earlier teachings rather than a unique system of thought originating with its author. It seems to be a distillation of the yogic knowledge of its time, a synthesis of diverse, even contradictory, traditions but deeply informed by the author's personal vision of realization. Both overarching realms of yogic endeavor, the liberatory and the magical, are acknowledged, although Patañjali firmly emphasizes the former. As one turns to earlier yogic texts or references, it becomes clear that some of the concepts found in the *Yoga-Sūtra* might well be the product of many centuries, indeed millennia, of experimentation, refinement, and philosophical contention.

Second, it is probable that Patañjali intended the *Yoga-Sūtra* as a guide for yogis under his tutelage, probably few of whom were literate. He structured the work as a *sūtra*, or "string," of 196 mnemonically condensed lines, to be memorized and perhaps chanted. In this concentrated form, unique to the Indian subcontinent at that time, the work is dense with technical terms and relatively free of verbs—a format particularly well served by the richly nuanced language of Sanskrit. One can imagine that it must have been as impenetrable to the uninitiated then as now, requiring considerable elaboration from a teacher. Thus, although there is broad agreement about the work's general themes, the meaning of its finer points is not always clear.

Finally, over the intervening centuries, several pandits have attempted to fill the need for elaboration by producing commentaries on the *Yoga-Sūtra*. The most famous and influential of these commentaries were written by brilliant ancient scholars affiliated with other schools of Indian thought. Though venerated and possessed of an undeniable authority, their interpretations are plagued by contradictions that have bewildered or misdirected many generations of scholars. Furthermore, they were written many centuries after Patañjali, their authors either unfamiliar or uncomfortable with his explicitly Buddhistic technical approach. Thus the early commentaries, so influential with all that have followed, betray little recognition of the complex way that the *Yoga-Sūtra* interweaves the contemplative approaches of the brahmanical-Upaniṣadic and Buddhist traditions with a *sāṃkhya*-flavored worldview. Nor should we expect them to. We today have the benefit of a panoramic historical perspective, fleshed out by a wealth of surviving texts that may well have been unavailable to pandits of the fifth or ninth century.

Despite these difficulties, there have been a number of first-rate efforts at interpretation in recent years, with approaches ranging from literal to poetic to devotional. As sympathetic as some of these have been, though, the complexity of the *Yoga-Sūtra,* as well as the obscurity of its roots, has a way of making the diametric goals of accessibility and precision frustratingly elusive.

Yet there is one more reason, perhaps the most compelling of all, why the *Yoga-Sūtra* can prove so difficult to absorb. Beyond its profusion of technical terms and also the seeming contradictions that have marked most commentaries, ancient or new, the greater barrier, by far, is that most readers have not traveled very far on the path to realization and therefore can relate to the *Yoga-Sūtra* only as philosophy instead of as a way of being in the world. This problem, coupled with the inconvenient fact that Patañjali begins with an elaborate and highly detailed discussion of the yogic end-states, immediately puts the work beyond the reach of many.

Thus it follows that most of the millions who today practice yoga worldwide are unfamiliar with even the basic concepts of the *Yoga-Sūtra*. Few are aware that, although many modern hatha yoga masters have tried to integrate it into their teachings, Patañjali's system predates the development of most hatha yoga by many centuries and offers a radically different program, primarily addressing the meditative approach to insight and liberation. And it is likely that a majority of those who have ventured into the *Yoga-Sūtra* were forced to turn away, thwarted by an impassable thicket of confusing jargon.

It is doubtful that Patañjali envisioned the *Yoga-Sūtra* as a stand-alone work, either philosophical treatise or yoga primer, for the general public. More likely he intended it for yogis in training, to provide concise reminders applicable to every area of contemporary yogic knowledge, including those domains in which he himself shows relatively less interest. Each line, itself also called a *sūtra*, might serve to jog the memory, impart a conceptual clarity to meditative insights, or provide guidance from that point forward to realization. That such resources might be helpful, even indispensable, at every point on the path is indicated by the central importance of *svādhyāya,* or independent self-study, in Patañjali's program.

It is also unlikely that Patañjali created the *Yoga-Sūtra* in isolation. He was probably an accomplished yogi with both deep personal realization and broad familiarity with the many strands of ancient yogic knowledge. There can be no doubt that he was literate and expressively gifted, having produced one of the great works of world literature. So, from all this one could infer that Patañjali might have been a celebrated and influential figure in his day, attracting large numbers of students from far afield. It is not difficult to imagine a scenario in which the great teacher, surrounded by dedicated students, might use a line or grouping from the *Yoga-Sūtra* as a starting point for discourse or practice. One can see how only the barest string of key terms, characteristic of the *sūtra* style, might be sufficient to set the most profound ideas in motion or to ease searching minds into tranquillity.

It is also easy to see how, after his death, such a format could eventually result in confusion. Because few observations are fleshed out very much, later translators and commentators have often struggled even with Patañjali's core themes. One can suppose that he would be surprised and disappointed by this, but it is possible that the *Yoga-Sūtra* inspired controversy even during his lifetime. After all, it presents a wide range of viewpoints, giving ample space both to the rarefied attainment of wisdom—*prajñā*—and to the worldly alchemy of yogic shamanism, perhaps to attract yogis of diverse sensibilities. And at certain points he does seem to be arguing against certain concepts of Buddhist idealism that were in circulation during the second and third centuries. Finally, some may have questioned whether the level of transcendent realization that Patañjali attempts to describe, and that he believes is unsurpassable, actually is the ultimate state of human knowledge. That these states exist beyond words and concepts, in fact beyond mind altogether, makes all such disputes difficult to arbitrate.

In any event, Patañjali's *Yoga-Sūtra* has come to be regarded as the definitive yogic perspective, or *darśana,* and has continued to serve as a primary practice resource for nearly two thousand years. Its durability and influence suggest that regardless of the way he balanced the disparate elements of the ancient yoga tradition, Patañjali's personal vision of realization has taken its place alongside that of Siddhartha Gautama, Buddha, as the most compelling yogic testimony of all time.

About This Translation

There are at least two possible approaches to rendering a work such as the *Yoga-Sūtra* in English. The first is to reproduce it in as close to a word-for-word format as possible, filling in the inevitable blanks where verbs, modifiers, or other parts of speech have been eschewed in accordance with the *sūtra* style of expression. This approach can best convey the highly technical quality of the work but makes for problematic English. The second approach is to find a more fluent way of expressing a line in English, which often means expanding it, perhaps substituting phrases, clauses, or even whole sentences for a single, highly nuanced Sanskrit term. Both approaches are valid and worthwhile; each conveys something the other cannot. Not without misgivings, I have chosen the latter path, ever attempting to avoid the needless sacrifice of precision for accessibility or vice versa. For example:

1.9 शब्दज्ञानानुपाती वस्तुशून्यो विकल्पः
śabda-jñānānupātī vastu-śūnyo vikalpaḥ

śabda = verbal
jñāna = knowledge
anupātī = following
vastu = object
śūnya = empty
vikalpaḥ = conceptualization

First approach
Conceptualization [is] following verbal knowledge, empty [of] object.

Second approach

Conceptualization is based on linguistic knowledge, not contact with real things.

There is also a choice to be made around certain Sanskrit terms—*samādhi,* for example—that may be regarded as especially technical or difficult but nonetheless essential to a basic understanding of the yogic tradition. Some authors have declined to translate *samādhi,* preferring to elaborate on its meaning in their commentaries. Others have turned to new coinages like Mircea Eliade's "enstasy," substituting a Greek arcanum for a Sanskrit one. Still others have decided on more familiar English words or phrases such as "concentration" (Aranya), "contemplative calm" (Miller), or "absorption in *Ātman*" (Prabhavananda). Again with misgivings, I have rejected the first two alternatives, although each has distinct virtues, in favor of the third, for example, using "integration" in the case of *samādhi.*

Arguably the most important term in all of the *Yoga-Sūtra* is *puruṣa,* which refers to the impersonal, unwavering awareness that underlies all conscious experience. Perhaps because *puruṣa* also carries the conventional meaning of "person," it has usually been rendered as "self," "spirit," "soul," or "seer." This is understandable, since most translators have assumed that Patañjali attributes a single, distinct *puruṣa* to each individual human being. Whether or not this is actually so, words like these tempt the reader irresistibly to personify *puruṣa.* Ironically, though, both Patañjali and *sāṃkhya* use this distinctly personal word to name the most utterly impersonal aspect of existence, pure awareness. The whole point of the *Yoga-Sūtra,* and of yoga—indeed, according to Patañjali, of life itself—is to grasp that *puruṣa* is separate and entirely different from everything else in nature. *Puruṣa* is just pure awareness, without any essence or entity behind it. A being and its consciousness actually are devoid of awareness; likewise, awareness lacks everything we might think of as constituting or belonging to a self. Patañjali states emphatically that the inability to see this fact *(avidyā)* is the central problem of human existence. Since he regards this as the paramount yogic insight, I have chosen "pure awareness" and "awareness" as the English equivalents of *puruṣa.*

While the *Yoga-Sūtra* is a culmination of centuries, perhaps millennia, of experimentation and fermentation in various practice traditions, it is a mistake to assume that Patañjali's terminology is consistent with earlier or later usages. The word *yoga,* as we have seen, means something quite different to him than to his predecessors, or to many today. Likewise, his uses of *ātman, āsana, prāṇāyāma,* and *īśvara* are all distinctive. This should not surprise us, though. When we today look back at an ancient tradition and its literature, we may tend to regard it as homogeneous and relatively consistent. It must be remembered that although we might group them together categorically, the surviving texts of yoga are chronologically and often linguistically at a considerable remove from each other, no less than Shakespeare's works are to us today.

I have also used the commentary to introduce and flesh out key Sanskrit terms like *samādhi* and *puruṣa* that have no English equivalents. In doing so I have adopted the convention of pluralizing the Sanskrit term where necessary with an *s,* as in *yogis.* This is not good Sanskrit but makes sense for the reader of English. And when such terms are mentioned, either in the commentary or in the afterword, "The *Yoga-Sūtra* Today," they are frequently given in both English and Sanskrit forms and also accompanied by a parenthesized reference locating them in the original text. It is acknowledged that this device, while helpful or even essential to some readers, might prove distracting to others. To the latter, my apologies, with the hope that this particular irritant can serve as a foundation upon which the pearl of compassion might form.

Lacking any wish or aptitude to engage in scholarly controversy, I must nonetheless acknowledge that this rendering of the *Yoga-Sūtra* of Patañjali departs at several points from traditional interpretation. The most salient difference will be found in the format of the commentary, which groups related *sūtras* together instead of providing a lengthy line-by-line exegesis. The latter approach is a hallmark of Indian tradition but tends to conceal the fact that the *sūtra* is a "thread" tying together sets of interconnecting ideas with rich collective meanings. Patañjali often requires several lines, probably meant to be recited and digested as a whole, to develop an important concept or technique.

In no way should this or any other departure from tradition be taken as a sign of disapproval, either for the ancient commentators such as Vyāsa and Vācaspati Miśra or for my contemporaries. Each version that I consulted in preparing this work provided a unique mixture of direction, motivation, and pleasure, as well as profounder respect for the ancient author known today as Patañjali. To all who have devoted themselves to the *Yoga-Sūtra,* I extend the deepest admiration and gratitude.

MORE ABOUT THE *YOGA-SŪTRA* ONLINE

In the interest of offering a print version of the *Yoga-Sūtra* that is accessible, precise, and not overwhelmed by scholarly material, all textual and translation materials have been made available online. Interested readers are directed to *www.arlingtoncenter.org/yoga sutra.html.*

From this site the *Yoga-Sūtra* can be viewed, downloaded, and printed as a PDF file. The text is offered in several formats: Sanskrit in *devanāgarī* script with alphabet and pronunciation guide; Sanskrit in transliterated roman lettering with diacritical marks; word-by-word Sanskrit-English translation; and a Sanskrit-English glossary containing every word that appears in the original text. A bibliography is also provided, including Sanskrit resources available on the Web. This online addendum is meant to facilitate the process of study and absorption, making it possible to read the lines in English exactly as they flow together in the original text, with selective interjections of commentary, and at the same time to follow alongside with the Sanskrit text. In this way the reader might come more fully to appreciate the extraordinary richness of Patañjali's language and the subtlety of his ideas.

Although this book and its related offerings are meant to help the reader follow the path of realization to its end, one must acknowledge that it is as difficult to do so alone from a book today as it was then. It is hoped that this work will clarify both the possibilities and the limitations of the *Yoga-Sūtra,* indeed, of all words, to bring about wisdom and the end of suffering. It will have succeeded in this only to the extent that it inspires the reader to action, and to stillness.

APPENDIX C

An Outline of the Yogic Path (Sādhana)

Aṣṭaṅga-yoga (2.29ff)

1. *Yamas* (external disciplines): clarify one's relationship to the world of people and objects

    ahiṁsā not harming

    satya truthfulness

    asteya not stealing

    brahmacarya impeccable behavior, including sexual

    aparigrahā not being acquisitive

2. *Niyamas* (internal disciplines): personal principles governing the process of realization

    śauca purification

    santoṣa contentment

    tapas intense discipline

    svādhyāya self-study

    īśvara-praṇidhāna dedication to the ideal of pure awareness

3. *Āsana* (sitting posture): cultivating profound physical steadiness and effortlessness in meditation

4. *Prāṇāyāma* (breath energy regulation): sustained observation and relaxation of all aspects of breathing, bringing about both a natural refinement of the respiratory process and bodymind tranquillity

5. *Pratyāhāra* (withdrawal of the senses): naturally occurring withdrawal from external sense objects as attention interiorizes

6. *Dhāraṇā* (concentration): locking attention on a single object/field

7. *Dhyāna* (absorption): all mental formations relating to an object/field

8. *Samādhi* (integration): sustained coalescence *(samāpatti)* of subject, object, and perceiving itself

Factors that compose the path to realization (1.20)

śraddhā faith →
vīrya energy →
smṛti mindfulness →
samādhi integration →
prajñā wisdom

Polarities of yogic will (1.12ff)

abhyāsa practice, effort to remain focused on the process of stilling (*nirodha*)
vairāgya nonreaction, effortlessness, nonattachment

Elements of yogic action (*kriyā-yoga,* 2.1ff)

tapas intense discipline
svādhyāya self-study
īśvara-praṇidhāna dedication to the ideal of pure awareness

Fundamental qualities of nature (*guṇas*)

sattva luminous, buoyant, aware, happy
tamas dark, massive, inertial, indifferent
rajas kinetic, restless, suffering

Patterns of consciousness (*citta-vṛtti,* 1.5ff)

right perception
misperception
conceptualization
deep sleep
remembering

Causes of suffering (*kleśas,* 2.3ff)

avidyā ignorance of the true nature of *prakṛti* and *puruṣa*
asmitā self-sense
rāga attachment
dveṣa aversion
abhiniveśā clinging to life

Neutralizing the causes of suffering (2.10ff)

gross form meditative absorption
subtle form tracing back to inception

Distractive barriers to stillness (1.30)

sickness
apathy
doubt

carelessness
laziness
sexual indulgence
delusion
lack of progress
inconstancy

Warning signs of distraction (1.31)
distress
depression
unsteady posture or breathing

Ways to develop tranquillity (1.32ff)
radiating friendliness, compassion, delight, and equanimity
pausing after exhalation
practicing mindfulness of perceptions
thinking luminous, sorrowless thoughts
focusing on things that do not inspire attachment
reflecting on insights from sleep and dreaming
becoming absorbed in any object

Stages of the stilling process (*nirodha,* 1.17ff)
samprajñāta cognitive, accompanied by analytical thinking, insight, bliss, or self-sense
asamprajñāta noncognitive

Levels of coalescence (*samāpatti,* 1.41ff)
savitarkā on gross objects, accompanied by thought
nirvitarkā on gross objects, beyond thought
savicāra on subtle objects, accompanied by insight
nirvicāra on subtle objects, beyond insight

Karmic effects of integration (*samādhi,* 1.46–51)
sabīja "bears seeds," leaving latent impressions (*saṃskāras*)
nirbīja "bears no seeds," leaving no latent impressions

Thresholds of realization

samāpatti/samādhi coalescence of object, subject, and perceiving (1.41ff)

saṃyama "perfect discipline" of concentration, absorption, and integration (3.4ff)

viveka/prajñā discrimination between pure awareness and nature (1.47ff, 2.26ff, 4.29)

dharma-meghaḥ-samādhi deconstruction of experience into irreducible forms (4.29)

kaivalya freedom from suffering, through the fully integrated knowledge that awareness is independent from nature (3.51, 3.56, 4.26)

Glossary of Sanskrit Terms

Each of the Sanskrit terms appearing in this book has been defined and indexed below. To make this glossary more accessible to readers unfamiliar with Sanskrit, terms have been transliterated to the Roman alphabet, rather than appearing in *devanāgarī* script, and compiled in Roman alphabetical order. The parenthetical references indicate where each Sanskrit term can be found in the text. To sound out Sanskrit words correctly, see the Sanskrit pronunciation guide on pages xvii–xviii.

A complete glossary of *Yoga-Sūtra* terms can be found at *www.arlingtoncenter.org/yogasutra.html.*

abhiniveśā self-preservation (2.3, 2.9)
abhyāsa practice, action, method (1.12, 1.13, 1.18, 1.32)
ahaṃkāra "I-maker," source of egoism; the sense that identification is occurring
ahimsā not harming (2.30, 2.35)
aṅgam limb, component (1.31, 3.7, 3.8)
anupātī following, relying upon
aparigrahā not being acquisitive (2.30, 2.39)

asamprajñāta without cognition
āsana posture (2.29, 2.46)
āśaya store, residuum
asmitā the sense of "I," egoism (1.17, 2.3, 2.6, 4.4)
asteya not stealing (2.30, 2.37)
avidyā lack of wisdom, ignorance of one's true nature (2.3, 2.4, 2.5, 2.24)
brāhma-vihāras heavenly abodes
brahmacarya celibacy, impeccable conduct (2.30, 2.38)
brahman universal matrix
buddhi perception, intelligence (4.21, 4.22)
cakra wheel, energy center (3.30)
caturtha fourth (2.51)
citta consciousness (1.2, 1.30, 1.33, 1.37, 2.54, 3.1, 3.9, 3.11, 3.12, 3.19, 3.35, 3.39, 4.4, 4.5, 4.15–18, 4.21, 4.23, 4.26)
darśana vision, perspective, systematic view, philosophy (1.30, 2.6, 2.41, 3.33)
dhāraṇā concentration (2.29, 2.53, 3.1)
dharma property, visible form, constituent form (3.13, 3.14, 3.46, 4.12, 4.29)
dhyānā meditative absorption (1.39, 2.11, 2.29, 3.2, 4.6)
duḥkha distress, pain, suffering (1.31, 1.33, 2.5, 2.8, 2.15, 2.16, 2.34)
dveṣa aversion (2.3, 2.8)
ekāgratā one-pointedness, focus (2.41, 3.11, 3.12)
guṇa fundamental quality of nature (1.16, 2.15, 2.19, 4.13, 4.32, 4.34)
indriya sensory apparatus (2.18, 2.41, 2.43, 2.54, 2.55, 3.13, 3.48)
īśvara divine ideal of pure awareness (1.23, 1.24, 2.1, 2.32, 2.45)
jiva individual
jñāna knowledge, insight (1.8, 1.9, 1.38, 1.42, 2.28, 3.16–19, 3.23, 3.26–29, 3.36, 3.53, 3.55, 4.31)

kaivalya emancipation, isolation of pure awareness (2.25, 3.51, 3.56, 4.26, 4.34)
karma action (1.24, 2.12, 3.23, 4.7, 4.30)
kleśa cause of suffering, corruption, hindrance, affliction, poison (1.24, 2.2, 2.3, 2.12, 2.13, 4.30)
kriyā action (2.1, 2.36, 2.18)
kṣaṇa moment (2.9, 2.52, 4.33)
liṅgadeha subtle body
mahā-videha great vow
manas mind (1.35, 2.53)
megha cloud, rain shower (4.29)
moha delusion
nāḍī energy channels
neti neti "not this, not this"
nirbīja seedless (1.51, 3.8)
nirodha stilling, cessation, restriction (1.2, 1.12, 1.51, 3.9)
nirvicāra not reflecting
nirvitarkā beyond thought
niyama internal discipline (2.29, 2.32)
pariṇāma transformation (2.15, 3.9, 3.11–13, 3.15, 3.16, 4.2, 4.14, 4.32, 4.33)
phalā fruit (2.14, 2.34, 2.36, 4.11)
prajñā wisdom (1.20, 1.48, 1.49, 2.27, 3.5)
prakṛti nature, phenomenal world (1.19, 4.2, 4.3)
prāṇa breath, energy
prāṇa-vāyu vital breath
prāṇāyāma breath regulation (2.29, 2.49)
praṇidhānā surrender, dedication (1.23, 2.1, 2.32, 2.45)
pratyāhāra withdrawal of the senses (2.29, 2.54)
pratyaya perception, thought, intention, representation (1.10, 1.18, 1.19, 2.20, 3.2, 3.12, 3.17, 3.19, 3.36, 4.27)
pravṛtti arising of activity (1.35, 3.26, 4.5)
puruṣa pure awareness (1.16, 1.24, 3.36, 3.50, 3.56, 4.18, 4.34)

rāga wanting, desire, passion, attachment (1.37, 2.3, 2.7)
rajas motion; a fundamental quality of nature, or *guṇa*
sabīja with seeds
sādhana path to realization (heading of chapter 2)
samādhi oneness, integration (1.20, 1.46, 1.51, 2.2, 2.29, 2.45, 3.3, 3.11, 3.38, 4.1, 4.29)
samāpatti coalescence, unified contemplation (1.41, 1.42, 2.47, 3.43)
sāṃkhya one of the six perspectives, or *darśanas*, of Indian thought
samprajñāta cognitive (1.17)
saṃskāra latent impression (1.18, 1.50, 2.15, 3.9, 3.10, 3.18, 4.9, 4.27)
saṃyama constraint, perfect discipline (3.4, 3.16, 3.17, 3.21, 3.22, 3.27, 3.36, 3.42, 3.43, 3.45, 3.48, 3.53)
saṃyoga coupling, union, association, mingling (2.17, 2.23, 2.25)
santoṣa contentment (2.32, 2.42)
sattva clarity, luminosity; a fundamental essence of nature, or *guṇa* (2.41, 3.36, 3.50, 3.56)
satya truthfulness, truth (2.30, 2.36)
śauca purity (2.32, 2.40)
savicāra reflecting
savitarkā with thought
smṛti memory, remembering; depth memory; mindfulness (1.6, 1.11, 1.20, 1.43, 4.9, 4.21)
śraddhā faith
śramana ascetic
sthira steady, stable
sukha happiness, ease
śūnyo empty (1.9, 1.43, 3.3, 4.34)
śūnyatā emptiness
sūtra thread; condensed mnemonic verse
svādhyāya self-study (2.1, 2.32, 2.44)

tamas mass, inertia; a fundamental quality of nature, or *guṇa*
tanmātra subtle primary experience of sound, form, odor, flavor, or feeling
tapas heat, intensity of discipline, austerity (2.1, 2.32, 2.43, 4.1)
tattva thusness, elemental quality, principle (1.32, 4.14)
tṛṣṇa thirst, craving
vairāgya dispassion, nonreaction, nonattachment (1.12, 1.15, 3.51)
vastu object, substance
vedanā feeling, tone
vibhūti extraordinary powers (3)
vicāra insight, reflection
vidyā seeing, wisdom
vikalpa conceptualization, imagination (1.9)
vīrya energy, vigor
viṣaya object (of experience)
viveka discrimination (2.26, 2.28, 3.53, 3.55, 4.26, 4.29)
vṛtti patternings, turnings, movements (1.2, 1.4, 1.5, 1.10, 1.41, 2.11, 2.15, 2.50, 3.44, 4.18)
yama external discipline (1.13)
yoga yoking, union (1.1, 1.2, 2.1, 2.28)

SELECTED BIBLIOGRAPHY

Deutsch, Eliot. *Advaita Vedanta: A Philosophical Reconstruction.* Honolulu: University of Hawaii Press, 1969.

Eliade, Mircea. *Patañjali and Yoga.* New York: Schocken, 1975.

———. *Yoga: Immortality and Freedom.* Princeton, N.J.: Princeton University Press, 1958/69.

Feuerstein, Georg. *The Yoga Tradition.* Prescott, Ariz.: Hohm Press, 1998.

Iyengar, B. K. S. *Light on Yoga.* New York: Schocken, 1966.

MacDonnell, Arthur. *A Practical Sanskrit Dictionary.* Oxford: Oxford University Press, 1924/91.

Radhakrishnan, Sarvepalli. *Indian Philosophy.* Vol. 2. Delhi: Oxford India Press, 1923/97.

Radhakrishnan, Sarvepalli, and Charles A. Moore. *Sourcebook in Indian Philosophy.* Princeton, N.J.: Princeton University Press, 1973.

Rahula, Walpola. *What the Buddha Taught.* New York: Grove Press, 1959/74.

Tandon, S. N. *A Re-appraisal of Patañjali's Yoga-Sutras in the Light of the Buddha's Teaching*. Igatpuri, India: Vipassana Research Institute, 1995.

Whicher, Ian. *The Integrity of the Yoga Darśana*. Albany, N.Y.: SUNY Press, 1998.

TRANSLATIONS

YB includes the *Yoga-Bhāsya,* a fifth-century commentary on the *Yoga-Sūtra* by Vyāsa.

TV includes the *Tattva-Vaiśāradī,* a ninth-century gloss on the *Yoga-Sūtra* and *Yoga-Bhāsya* by Vācaspati Miśra

Aranya, Swami Hariharananda. *Yoga Philosophy of Patañjali*. Albany, N.Y.: SUNY Press, 1983. *YB*

Arya, Pandit Usharbudh. *Yoga-Sūtras of Patañjali*. Vol. 1. Honesdale, Pa.: Himalayan Institute, 1986. *YB*

Bouanchaud, Bernard. *The Essence of Yoga: Reflections on the* Yoga Sutras *of Patañjali*. Portland, Ore.: Rudra Press, 1997.

Desikachar, T. K. V. *The Heart of Yoga*. Rochester, Vt.: Inner Traditions, 1995.

Feuerstein, Georg. *The* Yoga-Sūtra *of Patañjali*. Rochester, Vt.: Inner Traditions, 1989.

Houston, Vyaas. *The* Yoga Sūtra *Workbook*. Warwick, N.Y.: American Sanskrit Institute, 1995.

Iyengar, B. K. S. *Light on the Yoga Sūtras of Patañjali*. New York: HarperCollins, 1993.

Miller, Barbara Stoler. *Yoga: Discipline of Freedom*. New York: Bantam, 1996.

Prabhavananda, Swami, and Christopher Isherwood. *How to Know God: The Yoga Aphorisms of Patanjali*. New York: New American Library, 1953.

Prasada, Rama. *Patañjali's Yoga Sūtras*. New Delhi: Munshiram Manoharlal, 1988. *YB, TV*

Satchidananda, Swami. *The Yoga Sutras of Patanjali*. Yogaville, Va.: Integral Yoga, 1978/90.

Shearer, Alistair. *Effortless Being: The Yoga Sūtras of Patañjali*. London: Unwin, 1982.

Shyam, Swami. *Patañjali Yog Darshan*. Canada: Be All Publications, 1980.

Stiles, Mukunda. *Yoga Sutras of Patanjali*. Pune, India: International Academy of Ayurveda, 1998.

Taimni, I. K. *The Science of Yoga*. Madras: Theosophical Publishing House, 1961.

Vivekananda, Swami. *Raja-Yoga*. New York: Ramakrishna-Vivekananda Center, 1956.

SANSKRIT RESOURCES ONLINE

Capeller Sanskrit-English Dictionary:
http://www.uni-koeln.de/phil-fak/indologie/tamil/cap_search.html

Monier-Williams Sanskrit-English Dictionary:
http://www.uni-koeln.de/phil-fak/indologie/tamil/mwd_search.html

Directory of Sanskrit Resources:
http://www.classicyoga.org/directory/sanskrit-directory.html

Acknowledgments

This book could not have been written without the help and encouragement of countless others. In particular I am grateful for the support of my family, especially my children, Olivia and Toby. I am also in the debt of many professors, friends, and colleagues who extended a hand at some point on the long and winding road: Carol Nelson, Betty J. Ruth, Bonnie Katz, the late Sol Levine and Bob Ebert, Tim Murphy, Marty Kozloff, Jon Kabat-Zinn, Mark Bryan, Roger Paine, Bronwen Murphy, Stephen Cope, Andy Olendzki, Mu Soeng, Barbara Benagh, Eric Read, Punito, Mukunda Stiles, Darren Main, and Patricia Walden. Special thanks are due to Richard Miller, whose expansive comments always manage somehow to provoke thought and also to settle it.

I would also like to commend Shambhala, and in particular my editor, Dave O'Neal. For many years I have appreciated their integrity and support for the dharma, and I am now blessed by their belief in this book and by their expert advice.

Finally, no words can express the gratitude I feel for those teachers of yoga and dharma without whose practical guidance any understanding of the *Yoga-Sūtra* would have been impossible for me: Nöelle Perez-Christiaens, T. K. V. Desikachar, Larry Rosenberg, Jack Kornfield, Joseph Goldstein, Michele McDonald-Smith, Steven Smith, Jean Klein, and Vimala Thakar. I am also thankful to Georg Feuerstein, whose yogic scholarship has been especially helpful to me and so many others over the years; Vyaas Houston, whose Sanskrit courses and insightful translation have been an enormous inspiration; and the late Barbara Stoler Miller, whose lucid account of the *Yoga-Sūtra* arrived in my life at exactly the right moment and became the proximate cause for this undertaking.

INDEX

bodymind
  abhyāsa and, 6
  absence of movement, 73
  aversion and, 24
  cessation of, 76
  consciousness and, 2
  integration and, 18
  karma and, 9
  relaxation of, 16, 39–40
brahmacarya (behaving impeccably), 35
brahman (universal matrix), 2, 30, 88
brahmanical-Upanisadic tradition, 84
brain in modern science, 90–91
brāhma-vihāras ("heavenly abodes"), 14, 52
breathing and breath regulation *(prāṇāyāma)*
  Buddha's view, 84
  cessation of, 94
  distractions and, 13–14
  five vital breaths, 56
  in path to realization, 32, 40–43, 77
Buddha. *See* Siddhartha Gautama (Buddha)
buddha-dharma, 52, 73
buddhi (intelligence), 49, 57, 67, 77
Buddhist teaching. *See also darśana*
  dharma in, 66
  emptiness, 82
  "heavenly abodes," 14, 52
  matter, 50
  mind, 81
  and *Yoga-Sūtra* compared, 83–88

cakras ("wheels"), 54
caturtha ("fourth state"), 42
cessation. *See* stilling process *(nirodha)*
channels, 53, 54
childhood and infancy, 33, 63
citta. *See* consciousness *(citta)*
citta-vṛtti (patterns of consciousness)
  absorption and, 64
  as dharmas, 72, 73
  introduced, 2, 4
  suffering and, 24
clarity, xv, 15
coalescence *(samāpatti)*
  breathing and, 41–42
  eight limbs and, 32
  introduced, 2
  nonduality and, 82
  posture and, 37, 38–39
  as way of Seeing, 15–17, 18, 73
concentration *(dhāraṇā)*
  interiorization and, 13, 15
  introduced, 9
    eight limbs and, 32
  in "perfect discipline," 45–49
confusion *(moha)*, 86
consciousness *(citta)*. *See also citta-vṛtti;* "perfect discipline" *(saṃyama);* stilling process *(nirodha)*
  absorption and, 63–64
  dharma-meghah and, 70–71
  five patterns of, 2, 4
  freedom and, 68–69
  ignorance and, 22
  integration and, 15–17, 18
  jewel metaphor, xiii, 2, 15–16
  latent impressions and, 63–64
  make up, 3, 49–50
  as object, 43, 61
  posture and, 38
  during *pratyāhāra*, 13
  pure awareness and, xii–xiii, xv, 27, 67–68, 81
  transcendence of, 51
  visibility of, 28–29

spirit *(ātman),* 2, 88
spiritual teachers *(śramanas),* 52
steadiness *(sthira),* 37–38
stilling process *(nirodha)*
  breathing and, 40–41
  Buddha's view, 84
  coalescence and, 16–17
  consciousness and, 4
  interiorization and, 13
  introduced, xiii–xv, xiii–xvi, 1, 8–9
  practice and, 2, 5–6
subtle body *(lingadeha),* 65
suffering *(duḥkha)*
  Buddha's view, 85–87
  causes, 1, 21–26, 65, 78, 85–86
  described, xi, 75–76
  dharma-megha and, 73
  distractions and, 15
  effort and, 8, 39
  freedom from, 10, 64
  "great disembodiment" and, 58
  nirodha and, xv–xvi
  pervasiveness of, 95
  pure awareness and, xv
sukha (ease), 37–38
sūtras, 93

tamas (inertial quality of nature), 7, 23
tanmātras. See perception *(tanmātras)*
tapas (intensity), 36, 93, 95
teachers *(śramanas),* 52
thirst *(tṛṣṇā),* 85, 86
thoughts. *See also* consciousness *(citta)*
  coalescence and, 16
  discrimination and, 29
  and pure awareness compared, 80–81
  stilling process and, 8, 9
  thought form, 46, 76
  wholesome, 33–34
time
  nature and, 69
  perception of, xiv–xv
  scientific knowledge and, 91
  as successive moments *(kṣañas),* 58, 59, 70
  transformation and, 50, 66
"tortoise channel" *(kurma-nāḍī),* 53, 54
transformation
  from consciousness to pure awareness, 27–28
  of forms, 62–63
  of *guṇas,* 66–67
  integration, 48
  material, 50–51, 90
truth
  language and, 94
  of past and future, 66
  of perceptions, 4–5
  phenomenal world and, 26
  yamas and, 34

universal matrix *(brahman),* 2, 30, 88
Upaniṣadic tradition, 84, 87–88
Upaniṣads, 2

vairāgya. See nonreaction *(vairāgya)*
vedanā (feelings), 85
Vedantic concepts, 88
vibhūti ("extraordinary powers"), 45–59, 62
vidyā (seeing), xvi, 78, 87. *See also* ignorance *(avidyā)*
viṣaya (support of an object), 65
vṛtti. See citta-vṛtti (patterns of consciousness)
Vyāsa, 49

wanting *(rāga),* 85, 86–87

*A*BOUT THE AUTHOR

Chip Hartranft's work bridges the traditions of yoga and Buddhist meditation. He is the founding director of The Arlington Center, dedicated to the integration of yoga and dharma practice, and has taught a blend of movement and stillness to students in the Boston area since 1978. A student of yoga chiefly in the Krishnamacharya traditions, Chip has also practiced *vipassanā* meditation for many years. He leads annual retreats in the United States and abroad, blending yoga movement, breathwork, and mindfulness.

More information, including how to contact Chip Hartranft and The Arlington Center, can be found at *www.arlingtoncenter.org*

Shambhala Classics

Appreciate Your Life: The Essence of Zen Practice, by Taizan Maezumi Roshi.

The Art of Peace, by Morihei Ueshiba. Edited by John Stevens.

The Art of War, by Sun Tzu. Translated by the Denma Translation Group.

The Art of Worldly Wisdom, by Baltasar Gracián. Translated by Joseph Jacobs.

Awakening to the Tao, by Liu I-ming. Translated by Thomas Cleary.

Bodhisattva of Compassion: The Mystical Tradition of Kuan Yin, by John Blofeld.

The Book of Five Rings, by Miyamoto Musashi. Translated by Thomas Cleary.

The Book of Tea, by Kakuzo Okakura.

Breath by Breath: The Liberating Practice of Insight Meditation, by Larry Rosenberg.

Cutting Through Spiritual Materialism, by Chögyam Trungpa.

The Diamond Sutra and The Sutra of Hui-neng, translated by Wong Mou-lam and A. F. Price.

The Essential Teachings of Zen Master Hakuin, translated by Norman Waddell.

For the Benefit of All Beings, by H.H. the Dalai Lama. Translated by the Padmakara Translation Group.

The Great Path of Awakening, by Jamgön Kongtrül. Translated by Ken McLeod.

Insight Meditation: A Psychology of Freedom, by Joseph Goldstein.

The Japanese Art of War: Understanding the Culture of Strategy, by Thomas Cleary.

Kabbalah: The Way of the Jewish Mystic, by Perle Epstein.

Lovingkindness: The Revolutionary Art of Happiness, by Sharon Salzberg.

Meditations, by J. Krishnamurti.

Monkey: A Journey to the West, by David Kherdian.

The Myth of Freedom and the Way of Meditation, by Chögyam Trungpa.

Narrow Road to the Interior: And Other Writings, by Matsuo Bashō. Translated by Sam Hamill.

The Places That Scare You: A Guide to Fearlessness in Difficult Times, by Pema Chödrön.

The Rumi Collection: An Anthology of Translations of Mevlâna Jalâluddin Rumi, edited by Kabir Helminski.

Seeking the Heart of Wisdom: The Path of Insight Meditation, by Joseph Goldstein and Jack Kornfield.

Seven Taoist Masters: A Folk Novel of China, translated by Eva Wong.

Shambhala: The Sacred Path of the Warrior, by Chögyam Trungpa.

Siddhartha, by Hermann Hesse. Translated by Sherab Chödzin Kohn.

The Spiritual Teaching of Ramana Maharshi, by Ramana Maharshi.

Start Where You Are: A Guide to Compassionate Living, by Pema Chödrön.

T'ai Chi Classics, translated with commentary by Waysun Liao.

Tao Teh Ching, by Lao Tzu. Translated by John C. H. Wu.

The Taoist I Ching, by Liu I-ming. Translated by Thomas Cleary.

The Tibetan Book of the Dead: The Great Liberation through Hearing in the Bardo, translated with commentary by Francesca Fremantle and Chögyam Trungpa.

Training the Mind and Cultivating Loving-Kindness, by Chögyam Trungpa.

The Tree of Yoga, by B. K. S. Iyengar.

The Way of a Pilgrim and The Pilgrim Continues His Way, translated by Olga Savin.

The Way of the Bodhisattva, by Shantideva. Translated by the Padmakara Translation Group.

When Things Fall Apart: Heart Advice for Difficult Times, by Pema Chödrön.